WRITTEN BY 11 GLOBAL EMF RADIATION SPECIALISTS

HOLISTIC EMF PROTECTION MADE EASY

Practical solutions to safeguard
your home and loved ones
from the health risks of
radiation exposure

WRITTEN BY 11 GLOBAL EMF RADIATION SPECIALISTS

HOLISTIC EMF PROTECTION MADE EASY

Practical solutions to safeguard
your home and loved ones
from the health risks of
radiation exposure

FOREWORD BY PROFESSOR OLLE JOHANSSON

PATRICK VAN DER BURGHT | MARTIN LATINO | FARZAD NEJATPOUR
ALLEN CHENEY | JASON KING | NOURA OTHMAN | SAMIR DERRAR
MARCUS SCHLUSCHEN | BEATA RAKOWSKI | AZUL FERNANDEZ | DAVID LANGE

Copyright

By Patrick van der Burght, Martin Latino, Farzad Nejatpour, Allen Cheney, Jason R King, Noura Othman, Samir Derrar, Marcus Schluschen, Beata Rakowski, Azul Fernandez, David Lange

Holistic EMF Protection Made Easy: Practical solutions to safeguard your home and loved ones from the health risks of radiation exposure

1st Edition. 2024 v3.1
ASIN: B0CYTDDFCP (Amazon Kindle)
ISBN: 978-1-923223-06-6 (eBook)
ISBN: 978-1-923223-07-3 (Amazon Paperback)
ISBN: 978-1-923223-08-0 (Amazon Hardcover)
ISBN: 978-1-923223-09-7 (Ingram Spark) PAPERBACK
ISBN: 978-1-923223-10-3 (Ingram Spark) HARDCOVER
ISBN: ISBN: 978-1-923223-06-6 (Smashwords)

CONTACT THE AUTHORS:

www.holisticemfprotection.com

TRADEMARKS

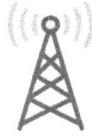

CONTENTS

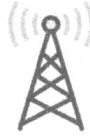

PREFACE

Welcome and congratulations on picking up this guide to better understand EMF radiation and how it can be investigated and mitigated in a way that fits into a suitable long-term approach to creating healthier living and sleeping environments.

This is a book co-authored by EMF radiation specialists from many countries. Whilst we have all taken a particular chapter and subjects to educate you, we can all assist with EMF home assessments. Doing things properly in the long-term has always been important to us and our detailed advice is based on a long history of benchmarking successes against the long-term outcomes for families.

The radiation subject can be confusing. There is so much misinformation around. People try to help their fellow men based on short personal experiences or hearsay, which is often incorrect and anyone can call themselves an EMF consultant—which, sadly, many people do with minimal or no professional training.

The internet is full of devices that will miraculously 'fix' your house or keep you safe, although no reduction in EMF radiation exposure can be demonstrated. At the same time, these products are advertised with a long list of research and awards that typically don't lead to real or relevant research or awards. This is all done to mislead people into quick purchases. Whilst the placebo effect can produce some improvement, it doesn't last when the exposure to EMF radiation doesn't actually reduce.

Then, there are verifiable solutions to EMF radiation that do reduce exposure and this is a good step in the right direction. What a lot of people forget, though, is that the end goal of dealing with radiation is to create a healthy environment. Not just a space with lower exposure to EMF radiation, but healthy *in general*. Also, dealing with one source or type of radiation and leaving others in place might cause a symptom to disappear but might not make for a healthier place to rest and repair. For this, we must look at EMF mitigation from a holistic perspective, in which we respect logic and long-term suitability from a health perspective.

It is important to realise where in our lives an investment to improve our situation is the most logical and would give us the biggest chance of achieving our health protection goals and enhancing recovery. Sleep is the most important time because that is when the body is supposed to rest and repair. Any money spent on improving your situation should start there. Without proper quality sleep, free of constant irritation, your body will have greater difficulty making significant improvements.

Whilst this is not a GEOVITAL book, the authors of this book all enjoyed training at the GEOVITAL Academy for Radiation Protection based in Austria. Having a unique background in working with patients, it was always important to have a holistic and long-term suitable approach to both assessing a family situation in their home and pioneering suitable solutions to deal with it. Doing things the right way, which is typically the long way round, doesn't often result in the cheapest solutions, but we think our health clients are worth it to do it right.

We are sometimes criticised for having more costly products by people who have never used them, or people who could not access them anymore after underhanded behaviour came to light. As a rule, those who have installed the solutions we recommend in their bedroom or home based on our experience of what works in practice are delighted with the effectiveness, long-term compatibility and results. That can't always be said for cheaper alternatives that anyone can access. We'd encourage you to make up your own mind and if you are considering the opinions of others, wonder why they focus on us instead of themselves.

This guide will help you gain a deeper understanding of EMF radiation, its sources, many handy tips you can use immediately and the logic behind investigating and mitigating it properly. Some authors will also have additional information available to you via downloads. In the introduction, we explain the logic of this book's flow.

Thank you for your purchase and if the information here has helped you, please tell others.

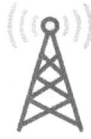

FOREWORD

During my whole work life as an academic scientist in the field of basic and applied neuroscience at the Karolinska Institute and the Royal Institute of Technology in Stockholm, Sweden, I have been taught that:

There are no bad, potentially dangerous, or stupid questions. Only bad, potentially dangerous, or stupid answers. Or lack thereof.

For many years, I have studied the health effects of wireless devices and technologies, such as cell phones, WiFi, and general wireless infrastructure. Decades ago, my research was instrumental in determining that the old CRT computer monitors were potentially biologically harmful and that is why we switched them out for the possibly less impactful flat-screen monitors. I also played a similar role in the protection of pregnant women in front of computers.

The simplest, and most common question in my own field of adverse health and biological effects of artificial electromagnetic fields (from sources such as cell phone systems, WiFi, tablets, laptops, high-frequency light bulbs, wireless smart meters, baby alarms, DECT phones, powerlines, smart cities, the Internet of Things and the Internet of Bodies, 5G, 6G, 7G, and much more) is from a parent asking: "Is this cell phone safe for my child?" Unfortunately, I can not say it is.

Neither can the world's insurance and reinsurance companies. These big players, like the WHO, the radiation protection authorities, the telecom manufacturers, and the telecom operators, are not naive, and they have, therefore - legally - all 'abandoned ship', some more than 20-30 years ago, leaving the consumers and their parliaments and governments completely behind on a ship that floats helplessly around. The big players' decisions are far more telling than any test tube, mice, or rat experiments I can show you, and it is therefore very high time to call these big players back. They sold us this current "safe" 5G ship, and now they need to prove that it actually is. And also for the other generations of phone networks, like 2G, 3G, and 4G, and the upcoming 6G and 7G, as well as for WiFi, powerfrequency magnetic fields, electric fields, etc.

Wireless communication is now being implemented in our daily lives in a very fast way. At the same time, it is becoming more and more obvious that exposure to electromagnetic fields may result in highly unwanted health effects. This has been demonstrated in a very large number of studies and includes cellular DNA damage (which may lead to the initiation of cancer as well as mutations that carry down generations), disruptions and alterations of cellular functions like increases in intracellular stimulatory pathways and calcium handling, disruption of tissue structures like the blood-brain barrier (which may allow toxins to enter the brain), impact on the vessel and immune functions, and loss of fertility.

It should be noted that we are not the only species in jeopardy. Practically all animals, plants, fungi, and bacteria may be at stake. For the latter, Taheri et al. (2017) have demonstrated that exposure to 900 MHz GSM mobile phone radiation and 2.4 GHz radiofrequency radiation emitted from common Wi-Fi routers made Listeria monocytogenes and Escherichia coli resistant to different antibiotics[58]. (Very similar results have recently been published regarding soil bacteria.) To say these findings are "scary" is a classical English understatement.

Because the effects are reproducibly observed and links to pathology can not be excluded, the Precautionary Principle should be in force in the implementation of this new technology within society. Therefore, policymakers should immediately strictly control exposure by defining biologically-based maximal exposure guidelines also taking into account long-term, non-thermal effects. This should include especially vulnerable groups, such as the elderly, the ill, the genetically and/or immunologically challenged, children and fetuses, indeed even egg cells and sperm cells (!), and persons with functional impairment (or rather functional variation/variability/diversity, as it should be correctly called) electrohypersensitivity.

Every generation of wireless technology also swells the ranks of these electrohypersensitive people who physically suffer from being exposed to electromagnetic radiation, whether or not they are aware of their electrohypersensitivity. Nocebo or psychological explanations are clearly not sufficient to explain the phenomenon. Electrohypersensitivity is a fully recognized functional impairment in Sweden, and therefore receives an annual governmental disability subsidy, and very recently it has also been officially recognized in the Netherlands.

Until revised exposure guidelines are developed, professional adults responsible for human lives in institutional or group settings, such as schools, offices, residential buildings, government buildings, hospitals, etc., should take heed of the large body of science showing serious risks and minimize these exposures at every opportunity by taking shielded hardwired approaches to, for instance, Internet and computer connectivity.

Science is providing ever more convincing evidence that the radiation emitted by our wireless telecommunications systems can affect biological systems, including humans, wildlife, plants, fungi, and bacteria. These biological effects are acting even at very low exposure levels.

The consequences on health and the environment can be all the more serious because:

- exposure is ubiquitous, repeated and/or prolonged,

- radiation from wireless technologies is modulated, pulsed, polarized,

- some individuals may be more vulnerable (fetuses, children, sick patients, people with preexisting conditions), and/or the effects may be much more prolonged (egg cells, sperm cells, fetuses, children),

- exposure is combined with other pollutants in our air, water, and food (e.g. chemical pollutants).

It is clearly not enough just to ensure exposure levels are below WHO-recommended levels. WHO recommendations are designed to protect cells from an excessive temperature increase successive to a single (!) maximal 30-minute exposure to radiofrequency/microwave radiations in an otherwise radiation-free environment—this is very far from reality. The bases for these recommendations were established in the late 1990s and have not been revised since then, even though:

- wireless technologies have developed very rapidly over the past 20-30 years,

- exposure pattern has completely changed (ubiquitous, repeated, prolonged exposure, exposure of children, fetuses, etc.)

- considerable scientific progress has been made in the identification of biological and health effects.

Not everyone agrees on the question of absolute proof of damage because a certain number of unknowns remain, even at the scientific level. However, there is no point in using the fact that not all the grey areas have yet been dispelled to assert that there would be no health and environmental effects caused by the widespread deployment of wireless devices and networks. This could even end badly from a legal point of view.

To date, we can no longer deny that thousands and thousands of studies indicate very real effects. The unbridled development of wireless systems is, in the more or less short-term, conflicting with the health and protection of ecosystems. Observations and return on experience indicate that damages are already in action.

I would like to remind you that, in 2011, the World Health Organization classified the radiofrequency and microwave emissions of wireless technologies as possible carcinogens, and 10 years earlier they had done the same with powerfrequency magnetic fields and their association with childhood leukemia. However, cancer is only one of the long-term consequences of prolonged exposure.

Radiofrequency radiation affects our cells long before possibly cancer develops.

Our body reacts with oxidative stress and inflammatory processes. When the exposure is repeated or prolonged, these mechanisms are maintained and may cause sleep disorders, disturbances in cognitive and reproductive functions, and damage to cells and DNA. In the long run, the body's defense systems are being exhausted and we increase the risk of:

- repeated infections,

- infertility,

- developmental disorders (e. g. embryonic),

- neurological and neuropsychiatric disorders,

- cardiovascular diseases,

- neurodegenerative diseases including Alzheimer's disease,

- cancers.

Egg cells, sperm cells, fetuses, and children are particularly affected because they may be more vulnerable, and/or the effects being much more prolonged. Also, they form the only basis for the future of mankind.

Against this background, it is a relief and reward to read the present book "Holistic EMF Protection Made Easy: Practical Solutions to Safeguard Your Home and Loved Ones from the Health Risks of Radiation Exposure" by Patrick van der Burght, Martin Latino, Farzad Nejatpour, Allen Cheney, Jason King, Noura Othman, Samir Derrar, Marcus Schluschen, Beata Rakowski, Azul Fernandez, and David Lange.

A book can not, formally, be regarded as a peer review-based scientific article, but with the authors' careful and accurate writing style, most of it could still pass as such. In this book, the focus is on our homes, but the general discussion easily applies also to workplaces, places of leisure, and public domains, like schools and hospitals.

The last years of research are covered, as well as some of the discussion around the functional impairment electrohypersensitivity. Metering/measurements of these fields, signals and general radiation are addressed both from a more professional aspect and also from what the layperson may be able to do using simpler handheld instruments.

As a reader, remember to pay attention to lessons about how to use and hold a meter and get familiar with what the values displayed on the meter mean to you and your family. All meters have tolerances in their accuracy and so a large enough safety zone or buffer should be maintained in an attempt to keep exposure well away from what, up to now, might have been demonstrated to be potentially harmful. More so when hoping to recover health. Also, mitigation measures, shielding etc. should be advised and guided by someone well-trained, and results should be verified. The book "Holistic EMF Protection Made Easy" points this out, but I would like to emphasize it once more.

Protection measures are presented, and several potentially powerful ways to introduce these into the home environment are summarized. As extras, you will find chapters about solar power and the construction, from the basics, of a - more or less - radiation-free home.

Of course, not everything in the book will appeal to every reader, and other experts in the above various areas may have details they would like to pinpoint differently, but it doesn't take anything from the overall current text - it stands well and firm on its own feet, no question about it.

To say that you ought to read "Holistic EMF Protection Made Easy" is too lame. I say you must read it, and act upon it after you have read it. And, please, note that one doesn't need to read every chapter; there is enough food for thought, chapter-by-chapter. So, if you have a special issue to address, use the book as a general reference text or encyclopedia, deep-diving into that particular chapter that is most relevant to your own needs.

If we do not engage now, we may certainly head towards a moment in history where future generations - if any - will ask us "Why didn't you react and act? You had books like **Holistic EMF Protection Made Easy** ... didn't you read it?!"

Stockholm May 23, 2024
Olle Johansson, Professor

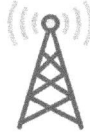

INTRODUCTION

In this guide, our authors—all EMF consultants—take you on a journey to a deeper understanding of EMF radiation. They explain what EMF radiation is, what research is available, what the sources are, and how to investigate it yourself or with the help of a professional. They also explain verifiable EMF protection options that fit into a holistic approach to dealing with this health risk. Also, they dive deeper into electrical systems and more complex wiring problems, as well as solar power systems considerations, how mattresses can burden a bedroom and the topic of Radiation-Free Building.

The book is set out fairly logically from problem to investigation to reducing exposure. To reduce doubling up on information, you may find references to other chapters to get more information on topics covered elsewhere in the book.

Research and EHS

Noura Othman, a pharmacist based in Egypt, explores the extensive research on EMF and highlights the inadequacy of the current legal limits to protect our health. She also explains the increasing phenomenon of Electromagnetic Hypersensitivity from public health and personal perspectives.

Sources of EMF Radiation

Martin Latino (USA) and David Lange (Australia) will increase your understanding and awareness of radiation sources, including transmission lines, local distribution lines, cables to and in your home, appliances, phone towers and wireless tech.

How to use an Amateur EMF Meter

Beata Rakowski from Canada explains what you should know and consider when buying and using an amateur EMF meter. Many people own an EMF meter, but only some know how to hold it, what limitations it may have, or what the numbers displayed actually mean. Beata covers all of this and takes you for a walk through and around the home.

The professional EMF Home Assessment

Samir Derrar from the UK explains what this book's authors can assist you with if you desire: the professional home assessment for EMF radiation. It is important to uncover and understand the complete radiation story that is going on in a home before investing in any mitigation. Assessing how the body is absorbing, especially radio frequency radiation, can reveal burdens that otherwise remain hidden. Some problems may be unfixable, in which case you want the ability to contemplate if you should not mitigate and strategise how to move to another home. In this chapter, you will also find the right questions to ask when determining if a person advertising themselves to be an EMF consultant is a good choice.

Little things you can do in your home right now to reduce EMF

Jason King from the USA has compiled many easy things you can do or consider regarding your EMF exposure from things in and around your home. He also elaborates on the use of cell phones.

Shielding radio frequency radiation with Shielding Paint

Marcus Schluschen from Canada takes you through the details regarding shielding paint. We do not encourage people to start shielding without proper consultation, but this chapter will show you that protecting yourself with shielding paint is not all that difficult once a proper strategy has been created. This chapter will also serve as a valuable guide for those about to apply shielding paint to protect their families.

Shielding radio- and low-frequency radiation by other means

Azul Fernandez, an Australian Engineer based in Italy, then covers the other solutions against radio frequency radiation and mitigation options that can be implemented against low-frequency radiation from electrical sources.

Electrical Wiring and Electrical Troubleshooting

Professional Engineer and Master Electrician Farzad Nejatpour from Canada explains electrical systems in homes using language the layperson can understand. He then discusses more complex situations that can cause magnetic fields that typically require an electrician to fix. This section suits those with rare problems and less experienced electricians who have been asked to help families mitigate these issues.

Solar Power done a safer way

Allen Cheney from Australia has a lot of hands-on experience with setting up solar power systems that produce a lot less of the typical EMF problems. Suitable for those wanting to install solar in a safer way or mitigate typical EMF problems in existing systems.

Mattresses and their link to EMF radiation and Health

Patrick van der Burght touches ever so briefly on an underestimated but important topic that should be taken seriously when aiming to create a health-supportive sleeping environment.

Radiation-Free Building for Lifestyle and Health

Patrick van der Burght, based in Australia, is one of the most experienced EMF consultant trainers and one of the few truly experienced consultants when it comes to radiation-free building. He shares important considerations that can save you in more ways than one.

At the end of each chapter, you will find a QR code to take you to the author or more information and possibly additional tools to download. We thank you for your purchase and trust this book will be a valuable guide with a logical approach to understanding and dealing with the EMF radiation risks in your life.

If you find this book helpful, then please do the following:

It took us months to compile this information for you, but you can help other families in minutes by drawing their attention to this book in conversation, on social media and by leaving an honest review on the website of your favourite online book retailer. Other people will appreciate it and so will we.

Thank you kindly and good luck on your journey of discovery.

Patrick, Martin, Farzad, Allen, Jason, Noura, Samir, Marcus, Beata, Azul and David.

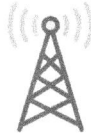

ABOUT THE AUTHORS

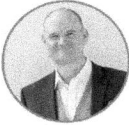

Patrick van der Burght
Radiation-Free Building Specialist, EMF Consultant Trainer since 2011, International Speaker, Entrepreneur

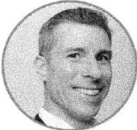

Martin Latino
EMF Radiation Specialist, Geobiologist, Entrepreneur, Abolitionist

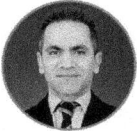

Farzad Nejatpour
Professional Engineer, Master Electrician, EMF Radiation Specialist, Entrepreneur

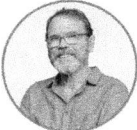

Allen Cheney
EMF Radiation Specialist, Geobiologist

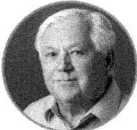

Jason R King
EMF Radiation Specialist

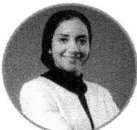

Noura Othman
Pharmacist, Health Coach, EMF Radiation Specialist

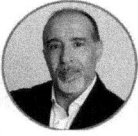

Samir Derrar
EMF Radiation Specialist, Coach

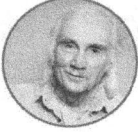

Marcus Schluschen
EMF Radiation Specialist, Geobiologist, Activist, Photographer

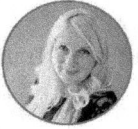

Beata Rakowski
EMF Radiation Specialist, Geobiologist, Activist, Polyglot

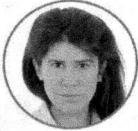

Azul Fernandez
Electrical and Sustainable Energy Engineer, EMF Radiation Specialist, Entrepreneur

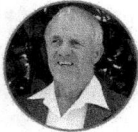

David Lange
Regenerative Farmer, Geobiologist, EMF Radiation Specialist

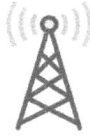

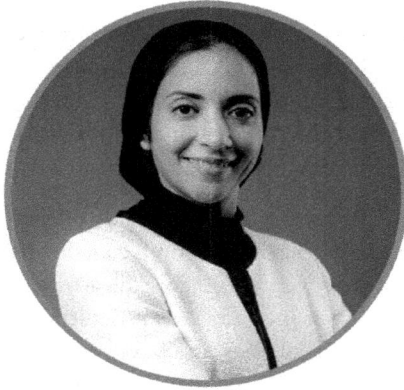

Noura Othman
Pharmacist, Health Coach,
EMF Radiation Specialist

ABOUT THE AUTHOR:
NOURA OTHMAN

Noura Othman is a pharmacist with a master's degree from Copenhagen University, specializing in disaster and crisis management. She held various positions at prestigious organizations such as the World Health Organization, Centers for Disease Control and Prevention, and the International Committee of the Red Cross. She discovered the world of electromagnetic fields through a deeply personal journey.

Initially seeking healing from the adverse health effects of harmful radiation exposure, Noura's own experience led her on a transformative path. Driven by a profound desire to assist those suffering from Electromagnetic Hypersensitivity and to support health-conscious individuals, she dedicated herself to studying and training as a geobiologist. Since 2019, Noura has been extending her expertise and services across the Middle East primarily in UAE and Egypt, offering invaluable guidance and support to those in need.

The experience of living with EHS can be incredibly challenging and isolating, especially in the early stages. Recognizing this, Noura places a high priority on building strong relationships with her audience. Her primary mission is to create awareness about harmful radiation and empower individuals to transform their homes into healthier living spaces.

Drawing from her journey as an electro-sensitive individual, Noura provides knowledge and support to help others manage their day-to-day activities and transition to a "new normal" lifestyle that is not only healthier but also practical and sustainable. You can find more about her work here: www.emfwhitezone.com

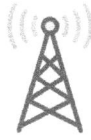

CHAPTER 1

RESEARCH ON EMF RADIATION, HEALTH RISKS AND EHS

By Noura Othman

Before encountering a severe case of Electromagnetic Hypersensitivity (EHS) in 2018, I lived a healthy life with a wonderful family and a successful career in emergency management. Despite my medical background, I was unaware of the potential dangers of EMFs until I experienced it personally. My journey to recovery was long and difficult, with progress that was not always linear. This chapter compiles the information and answers I wish I had at that time to educate myself and make informed decisions about my health.

In this chapter, I aim to shed some light on the scientific knowledge we have today regarding EMFs and explain the dilemma of the current exposure limits in place. This exposure can quietly affect us with minor symptoms like headaches, or build up in our systems to cause chronic conditions like infertility. With continuous exposure to EMFs, severe medical conditions can develop and, in some cases, become fatal.

I will also provide insights into EHS from both public health and personal perspectives. Whether you are personally affected by EMFs or simply a health-conscious individual seeking more knowledge on this topic, I have written this chapter with you in mind. I hope you find it useful, and that it helps you take one step further in your health-conscious journey.

Research Overview

History and Background

The use of electricity dates back thousands of years ago, with ancient Egyptians reportedly using the electric Nile catfish to treat migraines in 3100 BC[1]. Ancient Greeks also noted the concept of 'static electricity' when rubbing amber with fur[2]. History suggests that sickness from electricity is almost as old as its use. While several scientists in the mid-18th century were experimenting with electricity, the discovery of electricity is attributed to Benjamin Franklin, who provided a clear hypothesis and outlined specific conditions to produce electricity. Also, he was one of the first documented cases who suffered from electricity-related illness; in his writings in the 1750s, he was complaining to his doctor about *"a giddiness and a swimming in my head"*, *"a humming noise"* and, *"little faint twinkling lights"* that disturbed his vision[3].

"I do not doubt in my mind that, at present, the greatest polluting element in the earth's environment is the proliferation of electromagnetic fields" said Dr. Robert O. Becker (1923 – 2008), a researcher from the United States in Electro-medicine and is best known for his research in bio-cybernetics[4].

'EMFs' are harmful man-made radiations falling in the non-ionizing spectrum that can be divided into two main categories:

- **Low Frequency:** includes electric and magnetic fields resulting from electric appliances, concealed electric wiring, electric substations, high voltage power lines…etc.

- **Microwave or Radiofrequency:** resulting from using wireless technology and its infrastructure e.g. from cell phones, cell towers, WiFi, Bluetooth-powered gadgets…etc.

The exposure of the human race to Radiofrequency Radiation (RF) has exploded; it's estimated that, as of today, our exposure has increased a quintillion 'billion billion' times higher than natural background levels of RF[5].

This number is expected to exponentially increase with the adoption of the Internet of Things (IoT), the expansion in 5G and 6G cellular networks, and the proposed plan to cover the entire earth with a constellation of 10s of thousands of satellites[6]. Chapter 3 has more information about RF sources.

Growing evidence suggests that our exposure to harmful EMFs is making us sick. The World Health Organization has classified EMFs as 'Group 2B: possibly carcinogenic to humans'[7], the same classification as gasoline exhaust fumes. Thousands of peer-reviewed papers show the harmful effects resulting from our exposure to EMFs well below the currently established legal limits. Some of these papers can be accessed through The Bioinitiative Report,[8] which summarizes the results of almost **1800** studies predominantly indicating harm, and The EMF Portal,[9] which hosts an extensive database of **41,895** publications and **7,012** summaries covering the effects of EMFs.

Mechanism of Damage

EMFs harm human beings through several mechanisms. Three of these mechanisms include:

First: EMFs can interfere with our voltage-gated calcium channels present on the cell membrane, weakening them and allowing excess calcium to enter the cell. This can result in the formation of free radicals, which can attack our organs and systems, causing harm in many ways[10].

Second: EMFs can suppress the production of Melatonin, a crucial hormone with potent antioxidant abilities. This mechanism is associated with a high-risk factor in both the development of breast cancer and Alzheimer's disease[8].

Third: EMFs can disrupt the blood-brain barrier, our natural network designed to keep harmful substances away from the brain[8].

Health Effects

Some of the effects are mild and short-lived, like headaches, brain fog, itching, dizziness, and heart palpitations. Others are more serious and persist even in the absence of a direct source of radiation; for example:

- Cognitive disturbances and mental health issues such as anxiety, depression, and obsessive-compulsive disorder in adults[11].

- Also, exposure to EMFs has been reported to cause or exacerbate autism and behavioural disorders in children. [12]

- Weakening of the immune system, which leads to allergic and inflammatory responses, increasing the risk of many diseases and autoimmune conditions. [13]

- Reduced male and female fertility, accompanied by structural and functional damage to the reproductive system even at exposure levels as low as 3.4 microWatts/m^2, and carries on through generations[14].

- Cardiovascular effects[8].

- Development of Electromagnetic Hypersensitivity[8].

Many scientific papers have demonstrated the toxic and carcinogenic effects of EMFs, and I would like to highlight two major studies:

- **First**: a major 25 million USD study carried out by the US National Toxicology Program[15] found an association between exposure to **cell phone radiation** and the development of tumours in the hearts, brains, and adrenal glands of mice within only two years of exposure.

- **Second**: a study by the Ramazzini Institute[16] in Italy also found an increased risk of developing heart and brain tumours in mice upon exposure to **radiation from cell towers.**

EMFs' harmful effects are not limited to humans; wildlife also suffers! This has pushed some governments to take action; the Indian government banned the installation of cell towers near tigers' natural habitat and birds' flight paths [17]. The French courts ordered the shutdown of 4G antennas that severely affected the cows[18].

Bees have been observed to react negatively upon exposure to harmful EMFs[19] as well. One of the findings is that EMFs cause antibiotic resistance in bacteria[20], which is terrifying and aggravates an already existing global health concern. It's worth mentioning that these harmful effects occur well below safety standards levels set by governments around the world.

The compelling evidence of harm has led scientists to urge the WHO to upgrade the EMF carcinogenic classification to the higher 'Group 2A: probably carcinogenic to humans' level[21]. Scientists worldwide are calling for adopting lower exposure limits as seen in initiatives like the Seletun Statement and the International Commission on the Biological Effects of Electromagnetic Fields, which are two examples of the collective work that scientists are organizing to advocate for better health protection measures[22].

EMFs limits

It is only logical then to ask the question: What is a safe limit? How is our exposure to EMFs regulated?

Legal limits

Currently, there are no mandatory international regulations in place regarding safe exposure levels to EMFs. However, most countries[23] and organizations, including the World Health Organization, follow the guidelines established by the International Commission on Non-ionizing Radiation Protection (ICNIRP)[24]. These guidelines were initially developed in 1998 and have been minimally updated in 2020 for RF exposure[25]. They are primarily based on the 'thermal' effects of EMFs on the human tissues, which means that if the tissue does not heat up after being exposed to a single source of radiation for 6-30 minutes, it is considered safe!

There are several issues with these guidelines:

1. Long-term effects are not taken into consideration despite substantial scientific evidence of harm.

2. They don't regulate cumulative effects from multiple simultaneous sources, which is common in our modern lifestyle.

3. Vulnerable populations, such as Electromagnetic Hypersensitive individuals, children, and people with immunocompromised or neurodegenerative conditions, are not adequately protected.

4. They only focus on the 'intensity' and ignore the 'pulsation effect' of the emitted radiation, which doesn't accurately reflect the level of harm caused, as pulsed radiation is more biologically active than non-pulsed.

5. They exclude harm from non-thermal effects, which is a severe shortcoming due to the serious conditions[26] that develop below the 'thermal' threshold, as mentioned earlier.

In 2008[27], Professor Paolo Vecchia, then-chairman of ICNIRP, stated that these guidelines *"are not mandatory prescriptions for safety"*, *"not the last word on the issue"*, and *"they are not defensive walls for industry or others."*

Some mobile phone manuals mention the term Specific Absorption Rate (SAR) under safety settings, which is the value that corresponds to the relative amount of RF energy absorbed in the head of a user of a wireless handset and is expressed in Watts/kilograms. The methodology used to compute the SAR values by the phone manufacturers is not adequate to assess the health effects for various reasons[28]:

1. The tests are carried out on a plastic doll head called: Specific Anthropomorphic Mannequin (SAM) a relatively tall adult that doesn't represent the diversity of human body types. It is filled with a homogenous liquid that doesn't accurately mimic the complexity of the structure and the different tissue types present in the human brain, leading to different radiation behavior.

2. The testing methodology doesn't require the device to touch the body, which doesn't reflect real-world usage.

3. Only the highest SAR value is considered during the testing, which could be misleading. Let's consider this hypothetical example: Phone A is measured at 50 positions, and gives one reading at 10, 'let's assume at a position that is not frequently used' and all other readings at three. Phone B is measured at 50 positions, and gives all readings at seven and eight. Phone A will be labelled at a higher SAR value!

Although required by the US Federal Communications Committee (FCC) to be included for cell phones, the FCC states on its website that the difference in SAR values *"is an unreliable comparison of RF exposure to consumers, given the variables of individual use."*[29].

Health limits

There is a need to rethink the limits in a biological context. In response to this dire need, several organizations and institutions issued recommendations based on health effects relevant to our modern exposure and usage pattern, for example:

1. The European Academy for Environmental Medicine (EURO-PEAM)[30] issued guidelines based on a wealth of research papers, including the ones from the BioInitiative Report, that are thousands of times lower than ICNIRP. The guidelines also take into account the importance of distinguishing between daytime and nighttime limits as well as providing additional measures for sensitive populations.

   100 microWatts/m^2 is the limit set for **Radiofrequency radiation** exposure for the general public, which goes down to 1 microWatts/m^2 for sensitive populations. Compared to 20,000,000 microWatts/m^2 for general public exposure according to ICNIRP[25]. Some studies reported that exposure to as little as 6-128 microWatts/m^2 results in mental and cardiovascular problems[8].

The BioInitiative Report presented the different biological effects occurring at levels lower than the current RF legal standards in a color chart available on its website[31]. I include some examples at the end of this chapter for reference. Worth mentioning that Dr. Olle Johansson, an established authority in this field, suggests a far lower safety standard[32] at only 0.0000000001-0.0000000000001 microWatts/m².

2. GEOVITAL:[33] provides recommendations based on many years of experience in supporting patients with various health conditions. For **Magnetic fields** for example, GEOVITAL's recommended limit is ideally 0.3 milligauss to account for an adequate buffer zone, on the other hand, the ICNIRP limit is 2000 milligauss[34]. Researchers found that leukemia rates 'double' in children exposed to 4 milligauss.[35]

Some countries, like Russia, set their limits to protect against 'chronic' exposure to 'low' EMFs, which is common nowadays, therefore including non-thermal health effects as well.[36]

Other countries, like Switzerland[37], base their guidelines on the Precautionary Principle[38], using stricter measures than ICNIRP.

Way forward

The road to universal compulsory health limits on EMFs might still be long, but progress is steadily being made. Until this milestone is achieved, it's only wise to follow the Precautionary Principle to try to limit the scale of preventable morbidity and mortality that would be highly regretted but sadly irreversible down the road. Thomas Legge, ex-Chief Medical Inspector for industrial hygiene in Britain, said in 1934, *'Looking back in the light of present knowledge, it is impossible not to feel that opportunities for discovery and prevention of asbestos disease were badly missed.'*[39]

Asbestos was first mined in 1879 in Canada and people hailed the discovery and dubbed it the 'magic mineral' that contributed to the development of numerous products thanks to its unique industrial characteristics. In 1898, the first alarm was sounded to flag possible health hazards associated with its use. It was only fully banned from Europe in 2005[40] and from the USA in March 2024[41].

In 1895, the X-ray was invented and quickly became a popular form of entertainment at parties, as well as being used to measure children's feet in shoe stores. Carnival-goers even raced to have their hands and feet X-rayed. However, as with other discoveries, it took time for the regulation of X-ray usage to be implemented after evidence of harm emerged. Its association with higher cancer cases, especially among radiographers, became evident. In 1948-1950, trade union members gathered and decided that the exposure should be regulated according to the following criteria:

1. Justification

2. Optimization

3. (ALARA) principle, which stands for (As Low As Reasonably Achievable)[42].

The train has left the station, and it is only logical to think there is no going back to the pre-wireless world. Still, at the same time, there is no reason to believe that the EMFs will not follow the same general pattern of regulations of all newly discovered technology: wide use that leads to wide exposure, harm is discovered and documented, limits and laws are introduced and eventually endorsed and applied. As we no longer see X-ray machines used in street carnivals, one would hope that wireless technology will soon be used only when necessary. Some countries have already started this journey; France, for example, banned WiFi from kindergartens[43], and Belgium imposed restrictions on the use and advertisement of mobile phones for children.[44]

Electromagnetic Hypersensitivity

Humans didn't evolve to withstand so much radiation. We are bio-electric beings. Our cells communicate through electricity, and our nervous systems regulate our response to different stimuli through waves of an electric nature. The presence of external radiation interferes with our systems on many levels.

Medical Recognition

What if I told you that when a minority of physicians in the 1940s suggested that high blood pressure was a dangerous medical condition that needed to be treated, they were met with scepticism and even ignored by the majority of their colleagues?[45] Most doctors simply didn't believe there was such a thing as a 'high blood pressure' condition.

As our lifestyles change and evolve over the years, so do our sicknesses and diseases. There will always be a 'first time to hear this' moment. Well, Electromagnetic Hypersensitivity is no different. There is some resistance to accepting the presence of EHS in the medical community at the moment. However, EHS is now recognized as a functional impairment in several countries. The symptoms resulting from radiation exposure are given code W90 according to the International Classification of Diseases.[46] The American Academy of Environmental Medicine recommends that physicians start recognizing and assessing the total EMF load in the diagnosis and treatment of their patients[47].

The Emergence of EHS

Among the first reported cases of Electromagnetic Hypersensitivity appears to be the father of wireless communication principles and the inventor of alternating currents, Nikola Tesla (1856-1943). His biography mentioned that *"The ticking of a watch three rooms away sounded like the beat of hammers on an anvil"*.

"Ordinary speech sounded like thunderous pandemonium. The slightest touch had the mental effect of a tremendous blow. A beam of sunlight shining on him produced the effect of an internal explosion." [48]

The first group of cases, however, was reported during the 2nd World War among the soviet soldiers exposed to microwave radiation emitted by radars. The soldiers reported several symptoms, including fatigue, difficulty concentrating, emotional irritability, and cardiovascular conditions[49]. In the 1980s, Dr. Olle Johansson coined the term 'screen dermatitis', later named 'Electromagnetic Hypersensitivity'. In recent times, Gro Harlem

Brundtland, the former Prime Minister of Norway and former Director-General of the WHO, announced that she suffers from Electromagnetic Hypersensitivity.[50]

Public Health Burden

The estimate[51] of the prevalence of EHS varies between studies, from 0.7%-13.3, and up to 35% of the population if mild and moderate cases are to be included.

The onset and prognosis of the condition vary as well. It may start gradually with mild symptoms like dizziness, headaches, brain fog, skin redness, and heart palpitations upon radiation exposure and then may develop into a more severe condition. Alternatively, it can manifest as an aggressive reaction to any level of exposure to EMFs. If left without intervention, EHS can become debilitating.

There's still no definitive answer to why some people are more susceptible to radiation than others. However, one thing is true and agreed upon: prevalence is remarkably increasing and prompting the concern that one day, we may all fall on the EHS spectrum.[52]

A significant impact of EHS is the limited accessibility to office jobs; you need to work around being in an office with many WiFi routers, wireless printers, laptops, cell phones, energy-saving lights…etc.

Living with EHS

Identification challenge

All forms of sickness and diseases cause suffering and negatively impact our lives and the lives of those close to us. Still, there's an additional layer of suffering when one is impacted by a new condition not yet well-established in the medical field.

It's tiring and frustrating to get told that your labs and scans are all fine when, clearly, you are not! In my case, most doctors told me that there was nothing they could do to help me recover. It was frightening to think that I would be sick for the rest of my life. I also encountered some doctors who dismissed my claims and refused to read the research papers I had. (Yes, at

a certain point, I printed the papers and brought them with me to consultations). Some even advised me to stop reading and researching too much!

Reflecting on the early stages of my sickness, I now understand the doctors'
dismissive responses; they simply were not taught about EHS in medical
schools. Few doctors receive formal education related to treating EHS and
other environmental diseases. A study in Germany[53] found that doctors'
responses about the effects of EMFs *very often are not evidence-based and
might have major consequences in their patients' lives*".

Fortunately, medical guidelines for dealing with electricity-related illnesses
now exist. The Austrian Medical Association[54] and EUROPEAM[30] provide detailed guidelines for diagnosis and potential treatments. Functional
Magnetic Resonance Imaging (fMRI)[55] can reveal consistent abnormalities
in EHS brain scans, and Dr. Belpomme detailed the list of biomarkers[56]
needed to successfully identify EHS.

Healing Journey

Trying to heal myself was an overwhelming experience. Once I started
researching solutions, a Pandora's box opened with suggestions of things
to do, eat/not to eat, gadgets to buy, protocols to follow, and supplements
to consider…it was endless. I tried many approaches and healing modalities and travelled the world to attend courses and source my supplements. I
devised this formula to heal my EHS:

1. Stop the damage

2. Detox

3. Rebuild

4. Maintenance and boosters

I would organize all potential solutions according to the above formula to
build up my new routine. EHS symptoms manifest differently in each case,
some suffer from severe palpitations and skin reactions, and others report
the biggest burden to be on their nervous systems. If you scan the QR code,
you will get a full list of everything I tried and found helpful. But if there's

one thing I need to mention here, it's that there is a very slim chance that one can heal in the same environment that made him/her sick. We must ensure that we live, and most importantly 'sleep', in a radiation-free or at

Table 1

Examples of reported biological effects from exposure to Radio Frequency Radiation included in the BioInitiative Report		
Power density (microWatts/m²)	Biological Effects	Reference
50,000-10,0000	RF caused impaired nervous system activity.	Dumansky, 1974
10,000	RF affected function of the immune system.	Novoselova, 1999
10,000	RF induced pathological leakage of the blood-brain barrier.	Persson, 1997
2000-80000	RF caused a two-fold increase in leukemia in children.	Hocking, 1996
1680-10530	Irreversible infertility in mice after 5 generations of exposure to RF from an 'antenna park'.	Magras & Zenos, 1997
1300	RF from 3G cell towers decreased cognition, well-being.	Zwamborn, 2003
500-1000	RF linked to adverse neurological, cardio symptoms and cancer risk.	Khurana, 2010
60-100	Chronic exposure to base station RF (whole-body) in humans showed increased stress hormones; dopamine levels substantially decreased; higher levels of adrenaline and nor-adrenaline; dose-response seen; produced chronic physiological stress in cells even after 1.5 years.	Buchner, 2012
30-500	In children and adolescents (8-17 yrs) short-term exposure caused conduct problems in school.	Thomas, 2010
Legal Standard		Limit (microWatts/m²)
International Commission on Non-ionizing Radiation Protection (ICNIRP)		20,000,000
Federal Communication Committee (FCC) 800-900 MHz Federal Communication Committee (FCC) Personal Communications Services(PCS) public exposure		5,300,000-6,000,000 10,000,000

least radiation-safe environment. Sleep is when the body rests and regenerates. A naturally low radiation home is ideal, but if this is not feasible, shielding options are practical and effective alternatives when done properly. Chapters 7 and 8 have more details about shielding.

It helps a lot to be surrounded by supportive people when we are sick. We need help when we are vulnerable, and physiologically speaking, we need to keep our stress hormones as low as possible to allow our bodies to rest and heal. One night, when I was reading a bedtime story for my son, he said: *"I wish I could build you a city without radiation so that you can heal"*. It meant the world to me. In my healing journey, I was fortunate to come across doctors, scientists, and other EHS individuals, who were very supportive and exceptionally knowledgeable about EHS, I will be forever grateful for their kindness and I'm always happy to pay it forward to anyone who needs help with their healing journey.

CONNECT WITH ME

Noura Othman
Pharmacist, Health Coach, EMF Radiation Specialist

www.emfwhitezone.com

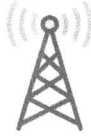

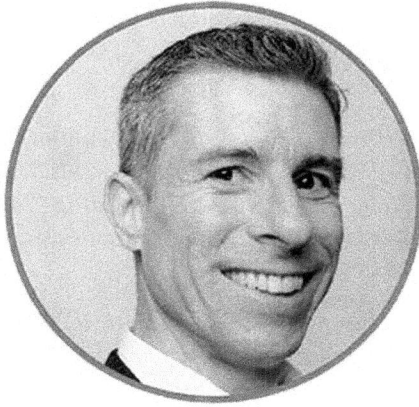

Martin Latino

EMF Radiation Specialist, Geobiologist,
Entrepreneur, Abolitionist

ABOUT THE AUTHOR: MARTIN LATINO

Martin E. Latino is a Professional EMF Consultant, Licensed Massage Therapist, entrepreneur, and former Electronics Engineering Technician. In 2000, he graduated from one of the most prestigious Technical Schools (E.E.T N°2 Paula Albarracin de Sarmiento), getting his diploma in Industrial Electronics, in Buenos Aires, Argentina. He currently lives in Central Florida.

Martin, founder and owner of Quantum EMF Solutions LLC, is a recognized authority in the United States for his innovative solutions to mitigate domestic radiation. He has been prominently featured in Healthy Living Healthy Planet and Natural Awakenings Magazines, for his contributions towards promoting healthy lifestyles and environmental sustainability.

In 2002, one of Martins' earliest experiences in EMI troubleshooting was from solving electromagnetic interference in churches and improving musical equipment. Along with his spouse, Deanna Latino, Martin ministers locally and nationally, seeking to serve Christ by sharing the Gospel and advocating for the defenseless.

In 2014, while running an electronics repair company, Martin became ill with an array of debilitating and inexplicable conditions. After exhausting conventional treatments, he decided to take control of his health management. In 2017 Martin leaned towards alternative approaches. He established his own company called Therapeutic Massage Services LLC, which focused on improving the well-being and enhancing the human body's internal repair processes.

In his pursuit of answers about the effects of electronic pollution on his health, he decided to study abroad in Austria at GEOVITAL, which has its roots as a naturopathic health clinic with four decades of history in radiation protection. As a Professional EMF Consultant, Martin was able to seamlessly merge the realms of EMF and the holistic wellness industry.

His desire to help individuals transform the quality of their lives has grown into Martins' crusade. As an EMF Specialist with a deep understanding of the detrimental effects of modern electromagnetic environments, Martin embarked on a mission to recreate healthier settings that help the human body thrive. He aims to work closely with functional medical doctors, chiropractors, electro-acupuncturists, reiki practitioners, kinesiologists, neurologists, athletes, homeowners, and realtors. He devised effective EMF shielding and building strategies gained overseas to significantly reduce patients' harmful exposure to electronic pollution.

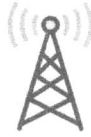

CHAPTER 2

SOURCES OF EMF - MAGNETIC AND ELECTRIC LOW-FREQUENCY RADIATION

By Martin Latino

Welcome! I'm so glad you are here! My desire is to provide helpful insights about magnetic and electric fields and how they impact our daily lives.

Since the 1920s, electronic pollution has increased by a staggering quintillion times, equivalent to a billion billion. Our bodies cannot perceive, touch, taste, smell, see, or hear it, but it can be very detrimental to all living beings. This is why it is crucial to understand all the different types of radiation and their sources.

In this chapter, you will learn about magnetic and electric fields from electric power, their characteristics, and their sources. I will briefly explain how these fields may affect us and cover dirty electricity. I will guide you through identifying sources of these types of EMFs, starting from outdoor areas and moving indoors, and then focusing on sources closest to your body as if you were holding a meter. I will advise you on what to prioritize when starting your journey towards EMF mitigation and improving your environment.

What are magnetic and electric fields - a brief overview

Electricity has been an indispensable part of our lives since the mid-20th century. I will predominantly explain the radiation that comes from it.

Virtually anything that uses electric power produces these types of radiation to some extent.

Electric fields are generated by the voltage in power cords and electrical wiring within the house. When a light fixture is plugged into a wall outlet, the cable gets energized, and this causes the cable to emit an electric field. The strength of an electric field is measured in units of volts per meter (V/m). Electric fields extend easily 2 meters or 6 feet away from their source. However, there are many ways to minimize their impact. Electric fields usually take the path of least resistance, similar to a water fountain that flows downwards toward the ground, which is something we can take advantage of. When the light fixture is turned ON, the movement of electrical charges (current) creates a magnetic field. The strength of a magnetic field is measured in units of gauss (G) or tesla (T).

The unit 'tesla' is widely accepted in the scientific community as an international standard. Depending on the situation, these fields can often be hard to shield against, and distance is often considered the best mitigation method.

This artificial radiation comes from anything electrical, e.g., transmission lines, power stations, power lines, electrical wiring in your house, extension cords, electrical equipment, or appliances. It can all produce this type of EMF radiation at some level.

That said, there is no need to panic and frantically move to a remote place. We can protect our families against EMF radiation very well by using logical thinking and a desire to make improvements that fit within a long-term approach to better health. You have more control over how you are affected by this than you might think. By reading this book and the information in this chapter, you will be a big step closer to taking matters into your own hands.

Electromagnetic spectrum overview

For individuals who learn better through visual aids, there is a helpful diagram known as The Electromagnetic Spectrum, which can assist in comprehending various forms of radiation. However, it should be noted that this is a very simplified explanation, as it only provides a perspective on the frequency of different sources alone. Signal characteristics, not just frequency, can create biological effects.

The electromagnetic spectrum ranges from low to high frequencies. The frequency of the field of radiation or a signal is measured in hertz (Hz), which describes the number of cycles that occur in one second. I will refer to extreme low-frequency (ELF), specifically power-frequency EMF, comprising electrical power.

Electricity in North America alternates at a frequency of 60 Hz, whereas in most parts of the world, the frequency of electric power is 50 Hz.

Electric and magnetic fields from electric power are not coupled, as they are at higher frequencies used for carrying information. Information-carrying waves are considered electromagnetic waves and will be covered in Chapter 3.

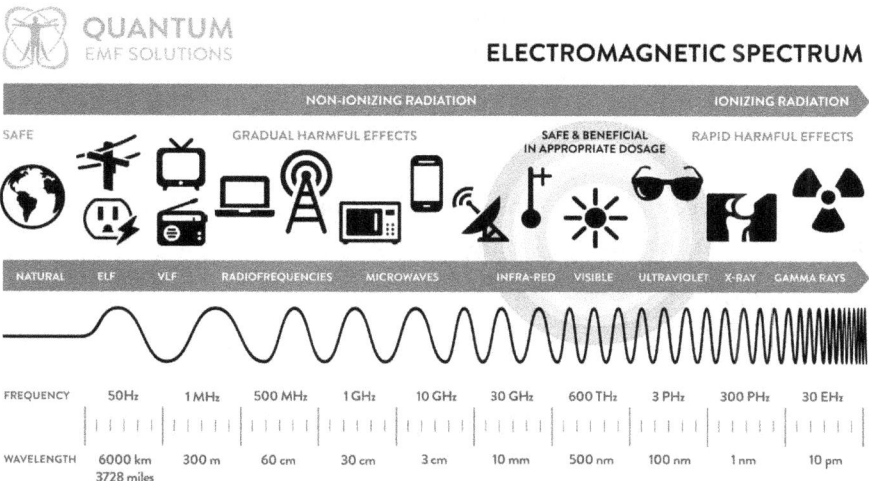

QUANTUM
EMF SOLUTIONS

ELECTROMAGNETIC SPECTRUM

NON-IONIZING RADIATION		IONIZING RADIATION
SAFE	GRADUAL HARMFUL EFFECTS	SAFE & BENEFICIAL IN APPROPRIATE DOSAGE RAPID HARMFUL EFFECTS

NATURAL	ELF	VLF	RADIOFREQUENCIES	MICROWAVES	INFRA-RED	VISIBLE	ULTRAVIOLET	X-RAY	GAMMA RAYS

FREQUENCY	50Hz	1 MHz	500 MHz	1 GHz	10 GHz	30 GHz	600 THz	3 PHz	300 PHz	30 EHz
WAVELENGTH	6000 km 3728 miles	300 m	60 cm	30 cm	3 cm	10 mm	500 nm	100 nm	1 nm	10 pm

Besides power-frequency, radio frequency and microwaves are all considered non-ionizing radiation. Although non-ionizing radiation may appear harmless, it can gradually and subtly affect us over time. Epidemiological studies consistently link potential EMF exposure to increased risk of childhood leukemia and much more.

Magnetic Fields Sources:

Let me take you on a little journey to consider the sources of magnetic fields in and around the home. We will imagine we're standing outside and we are walking towards the bedroom.

Transmission lines

High-voltage transmission lines, also known as Pylons or Walkers, are designed to transmit electricity over long distances. The magnetic fields generated by these lines are strong and can extend a fair distance from the lines themselves, and sadly, people are allowed to build or purchase homes too close to these structures.

Power lines (local distribution lines)

You have likely never thought about the power lines running along your street. They, too, can throw off harmful magnetic fields. Above-ground power lines tend to produce stronger fields because their cables are separated. Having the power cables on your side of the street places you closer to this potential problem.

Transformers

Have you ever come across those barrels or boxes that are suspended from power lines on the streets? Or those big boxes standing between homes? They can produce strong magnetic fields as well. Some are relatively weak, but others can reach far into homes.

Get a meter and you'll know

Shielding against magnetic fields is costly and often results in disappointment when utilized in a residential setting. Therefore, it's important to avoid buying or renting homes too close to transmission lines or any other electrical hardware that produces strong magnetic fields that reach into homes. It is critical to assess the magnetic fields inside any home, but especially near transmission lines, power lines, and transformers. If you would like to learn how to use an amateur EMF meter read Chapter 4.

Diurnal cycle

The magnetic fields emitted by transmission lines and street power lines may vary during the day due to changes in power consumption.

The highest exposure typically occurs between 3 PM and 10 PM. From 10 PM to 7 AM, the exposure levels tend to be the lowest, and from 7 AM to 3 PM, the levels are usually moderate. Ideally, you would want your exposure to stay below the recommended maximums outlined in Chapter 4.

How close is too close?

When it comes to the magnetic fields from electrical installations, people often ask: What is a safe distance? There is no easy answer. The amount of magnetic fields produced depends on many factors, such as the amount of electricity being carried, the proper balance between the cables, etc.

Whichever distance figure I gave to the 'safe distance question', I would be doing you a disservice. If I were conservative, I would steer you to exclude homes that might be perfectly fine. If I weren't conservative enough, I would lead you to determine that homes would be safe when they might not be. The simple answer to this is to take a meter on-site and take readings so you know what the exposure is and take action from there.

As we 'walk' closer to the house we can possibly see solar panels. Let's talk about them. Photovoltaic panels, inverters, circuit breaker panels, and meter boxes, can all produce magnetic fields that reach into the home.

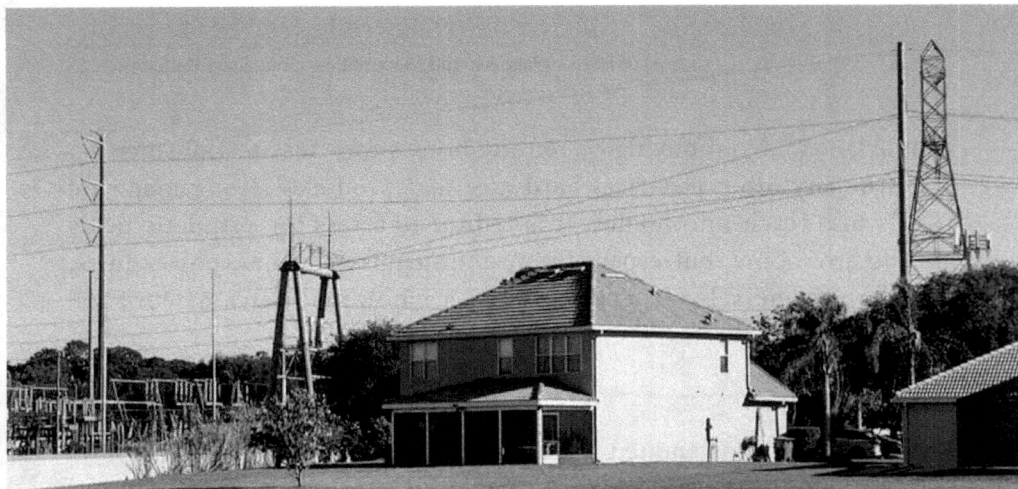

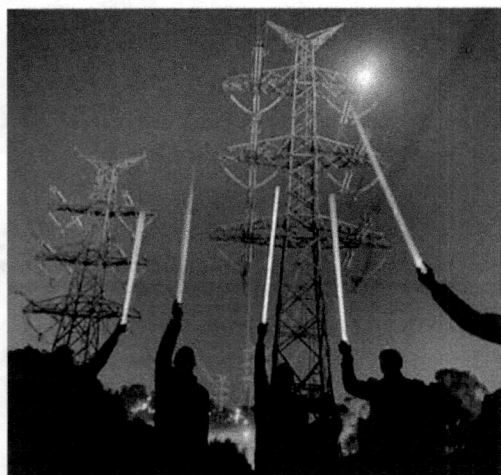

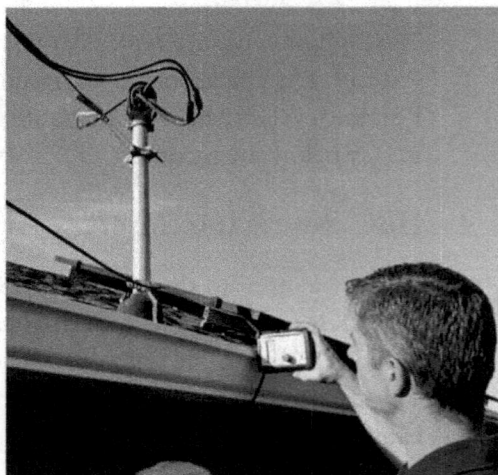

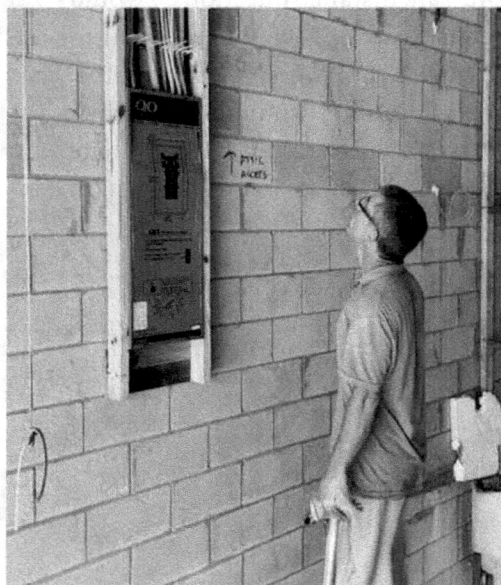

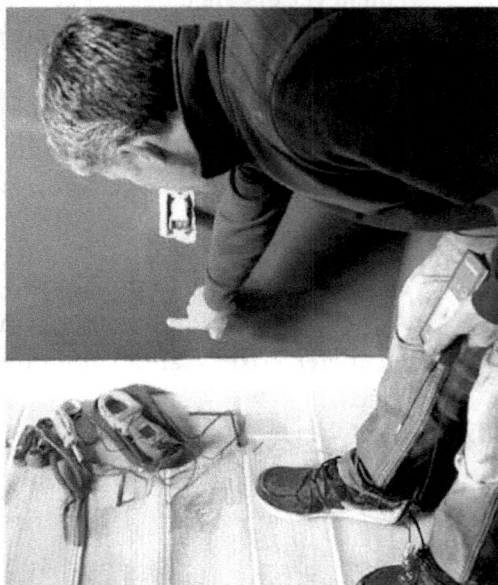

Solar power systems, breaker panel, and the meter box

Some solar power systems can produce strong magnetic fields, but others are fairly weak. The same with the inverters. The good news is, at night, during sleep, they don't do anything. Chapter 10 is dedicated to solar power. Circuit breaker panels and utility meters are often places that produce magnetic fields. Typically, they are not strong, but strong enough to disturb sleep and possibly affect your health if they are located on a bedroom wall. Magnetic fields are common here because the hot/active/live power cable and the neutral are separated. The separation produces some magnetic fields.

Stray current

In brief, stray current is when electrical current is lost by other properties and travels over the soil or often copper water pipes, and tracks through other homes to return to the power lines in the street. The result is that you have a much stronger magnetic field around your circuit breaker panel, the cables connecting to the street power, and the cable connecting your home to the ground. More in Chapter 9.

Wiring errors

Wiring errors are not so common but do seem to be more likely caused by unqualified electricians. The current going out into an electrical circuit of the home should come back on the same path. A wiring error occurs when the returning current is able to take an alternative path due to an incorrect connection. The results are intense magnetic fields in the home when power is used on that circuit. Chapter 4 touches on this, and is covered in great detail in Chapter 9.

If you find significant magnetic fields in the home, it is best to seek the guidance of a professional EMF Consultant.

Electric vehicles

People are considering going green by buying electric vehicles. Electric vehicles do tend to produce more EMF exposure than conventional cars, but inevitably we need to go electric for the environment. People don't consider that in-house charging stations require a lot of electricity. The associated hardware can cause magnetic and electric field exposure.

Magnetic fields in living spaces

We've arrived inside where many of our appliances produce magnetic fields, but most of those are insignificant. The importance of the bedroom for health protection and restoration is higher than daytime exposure. However, reducing daytime exposure is still beneficial. In the daytime, it is important to focus on things that affect the areas where you spend a lot of time.

Here are the more important ones to look out for:

LIVING ROOM	KITCHEN	OFFICE
Behind the fuse/panel box	Electric stove	Chargers & Adapters
Adjustable chairs	Range hood/fan	Laptops close to body
Near electric car charger	Refrigerators	Pedestal/ tower/ desk fans
Electric floor heating	Air fryers	Air purifiers
Space heaters	Blenders/mixers	Window air conditioning units

Some other items you might not have considered

Hair dryers can create a strong magnetic field. If you are a hairdresser, it would be a concern.

Older tube TVs can produce magnetic fields up to 6 feet (2 meters) in diameter. However, modern flat TVs are typically fine in terms of magnetic fields. On the other hand, they emit high-frequency radiation, which could be a concern.

It is important to note that placing laptops on your lap is not recommended, not only because of ergonomics but also because these fields can penetrate almost any surface and cause potential harm to reproductive organs.

Saunas and exercise equipment can generate magnetic and electric fields. However, this might be considered less of a problem because they are used for a short time and such equipment can provide significant health benefits.

Magnetic field sources in the bedroom

It is crucial to address the presence of magnetic fields and other sources of EMF radiation in bedrooms. The logic is simple: Our body repairs itself almost exclusively during sleep. Your body functions on very subtle electrical signals, and we can't expect our body to function optimally if we are constantly irritated by man-made signals.

It is unfortunate when homes have their utility meter and/or circuit breaker panels installed on bedroom walls. Consider arranging your headboard on a different wall.

Various devices such as alarm clocks, wireless cell phone charging stations, space heaters, and adjustable bed frames can generate magnetic fields that reach the body in a bedroom. The use of electrical heating pads or blankets can also create these fields and has been linked to fetal growth defects and miscarriages. (Wertheimer and Leeper, 1986)

Static magnetic fields produced by metal springs inside the mattress or spring box can also be problematic since they are near the body. As described in Chapter 11, a compass can be used to check for the presence of these fields.

Electric Fields Sources:

Now that we have reached the bedroom in our little virtual walk, let's switch gears, discuss electric fields in the bedroom, and then move outdoors.

Electric fields are caused by the presence of voltage in power cables, house wiring, appliances, and everything in between. Their strength increases proportionately with the voltage.

This form of alternating electrical power is something that has never existed in nature, and our bodies don't know how to process it. Our nervous system and bodies have been created to work on direct current.

As long as voltage is present, electric fields will be generated, so even if the equipment is turned off but is still connected to the source of electric power, the electric fields will remain. Even if we unplug everything in a home, the wiring in the walls still emits electric fields in great quantities.

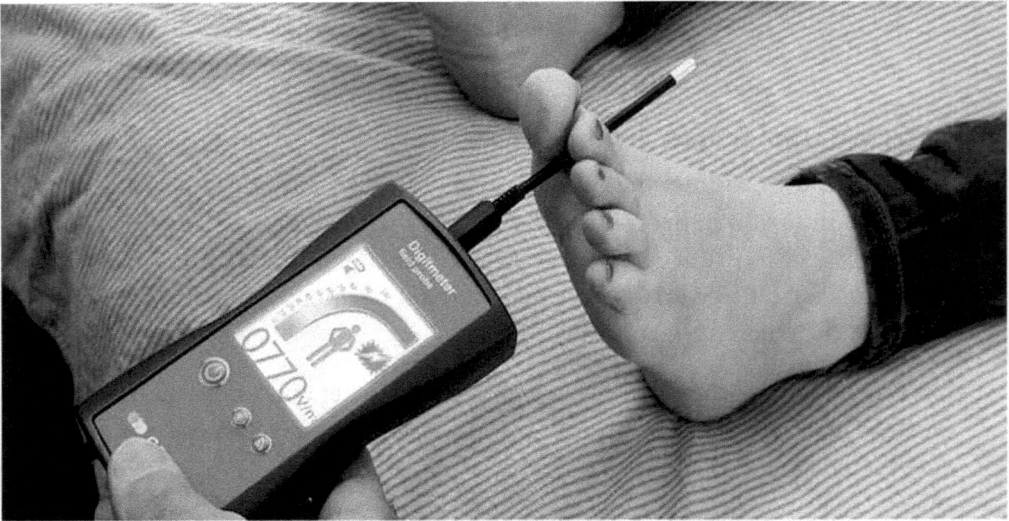

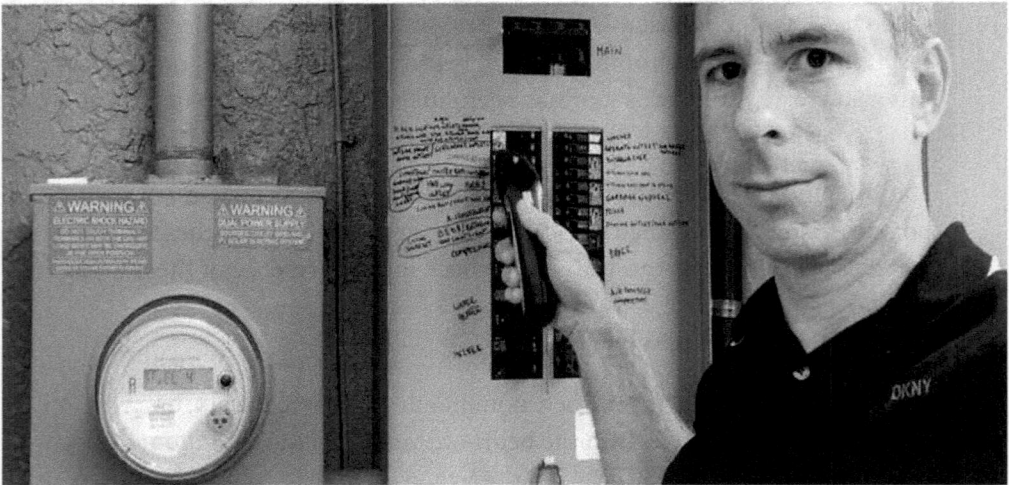

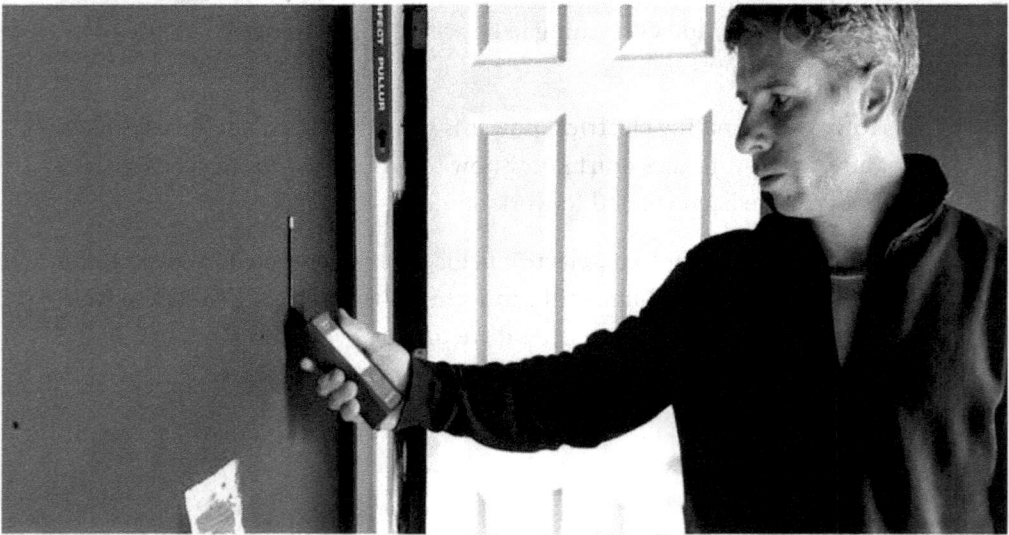

Electric field sources in the bedroom

Addressing electric fields is crucial to create a healthy bedroom. Ignoring them is not an option as they are an important piece of the puzzle.

Similar to magnetic fields, these electric fields will come from heating blankets or heating pads. Electric adjustable beds connected to power will produce electric fields, especially if the frame is metal. Electric fields can be aggravated with a standard spring mattress or box spring, which inadvertently increases EMF.

Electric fields will come from your bedside table lamp, alarm clocks connected to wall outlets, cellphone chargers, extension cords under the bed, and space heaters.

As mentioned, electric fields can easily extend 2 meters or 6 feet from their source, engulfing us 50 or 60 times per second! In our experience, 95% of people have this excessive exposure in the bedroom.

There are a lot of recommendations online about shutting off circuit breakers to eliminate electrical power going to your bedroom. I must warn you that circuit breakers are not light switches; they can be awkward and hazardous. See Chapter 5.

Electrical power supply cables running past the bedroom sometimes steer mitigation in different directions. See Chapter 8.

Electric fields in living spaces and office

With our homes completely electrified, there is wiring and voltage around you nearly everywhere, so it is exceedingly tricky to find a space without this exposure in existing homes. In newly built homes, much can be done to avoid this. See Chapter 12.

Every electrical cable plugged into outlets and their appliances will push more electric fields into your living spaces. Here are a few things that may warrant particular attention:

- Chairs plugged into electricity for motorized adjustment or other reasons
- Extension cords placed behind sofas
- Electric floor heating
- Radiant heating panels
- Solar panel and equipment
- Metal desk

In the home office, it is hard not to be exposed to more electric fields from everything we plug in. Our answer is: Unplug what you don't need all the time. A metal desk can make exposure worse.

Electric fields outside

Stepping outside the home, power lines in the street or transmission lines will have electric fields 'pouring' off them. If you or the children spend significant time in the front yard, this exposure is clearly not desired.

If power or transmission lines are close enough to pour electric fields on you, they will also expose you to magnetic fields, and depending on your exposure, you may not want to be there long-term.

That said, electric fields want to go to the ground, and if moving is not an option or you want to reduce your exposure to electric fields, then you could plant some fast-growing trees on the property line that will grow into an electric field barrier and reduce your exposure. In the same way, a pergola with a creeper growing over it will offer similar protection for sitting underneath it.

What is Dirty Electricity?

To properly understand what dirty electricity is, it is vital first to comprehend the fundamental attributes of electricity.

Electricity is composed of many factors and can be represented by a sine wave. The sine wave of a smooth alternating current (AC) is like a slow breeze moving across the surface of a lake, creating ripples in the water.

Electric utilities or power companies provide AC at a frequency of 50 or 60 Hertz (cycles per second).

Dirty electricity is a form of electrical pollution. It is also known as electromagnetic interference, line noise, or harmonic transients. This noise is a high-frequency transient above 1.5 KHz. When noise is introduced, it will converge, couple, and ride along the sine wave the power company provides, resembling turbulent waters.

What creates dirty electricity?

This type of electrical pollution is caused by changes in the quality of electricity by arcing, sparking, and any device interrupting the current flow repeatedly, often thousands of times per second. This phenomenon is also sometimes observed in modern devices needing to comply with governmental standards.

Dirty electricity is a common issue in many homes. While the power may be 'clean' when it comes out of the power plant, it often becomes contaminated with unwanted transients when it reaches your house.

Many solar power installations can also produce line noise, and when you have some of those in your street, what they push into the grid will come into your home even if you don't have solar yourself or opted out of a smart meter. Refer to Chapter 10 about Solar power and DE.

Here is a list of some of the most common producers of dirty electricity:

Air Conditioning Units	Multi-speed Fans
Battery chargers	Refrigerators
Blenders and mixers	Smart meters
Cordless phones	Street lights
Fluorescent lightbulbs & tubes	Switching power adapters
Hair Dryers	Solar panel systems

LED light bulbs	Televisions
LED strips	Transmission lines or Pylons
Light dimmer switches	Video game consoles
Microwave ovens	Wi-Fi routers and modems

Dirty electricity filters pros and cons:

Filters are available to reduce this 'noise' that can be present in the electricity. The argument against using these filters is that the motivation to buy filters typically comes from meters you plug into a socket that gives you a number. Based on this number, people selling filters will urge you to buy more and keep buying them till the number is below a certain value they recommend.

A 'number' from a plug-in meter doesn't necessarily convey the radiation that comes into the living space in quantities worth prioritizing. When we assess the space inside the room, the presence of DE can often not be very convincing. When levels are high, clearly, there is a problem that may need to be addressed, but in terms of priorities, I put DE filters that may complement the approach of creating a healthy bedroom as a last thing.

Plug-in dirty electricity filters can clean your power to some extent, depending on the situation, but they completely ignore the presence of magnetic fields, radio frequency radiation, and electric fields in the home and, more importantly, the bedroom. When we address the burdens in the bedroom, DE is often also addressed as we tend to cut the power to circuits whose electric fields bother the sleeper. If you do that with relays that cut both the hot/active and the neutral, there can be no DE transmitted from those circuits either.

These filters are also a double-edged sword. It is not advisable to use them if you have socket wiring issues or household electricity loops. On certain occasions, these plug-in DE filters have been reported to have damaged solar power inverters. Also, in some situations, sensitive (EHS) people have found it not to be beneficial for them or made their symptoms worse.

Don't get me wrong—these plugin filters work well for what they are intended to do, but there is a lot to consider before plugging these filters into your home's outlets. Yes, dirty electricity is an issue we recognize; it can be investigated, but we prioritize removing 'all' interference from the bedroom.

Final Thoughts

Congratulations on having the interest to find out more about what might be affecting your life and loved ones! I trust this chapter provided you with a better understanding of the electrical space around you and helped you take action in your home.

Our specialized services are designed to tackle these issues head-on, providing you with understanding, a logical long-term approach to a healthier home and having the peace of mind knowing your home is protected.

I share valuable things for you to download. If you follow the link in the QR code provided, you will also have the ability to connect with me.

CONNECT WITH ME

Martin Latino

EMF Radiation Specialist, Geobiologist, Entrepreneur, Abolitionist

https://quantumemfsolutions.com/bookbonus/

David Lange

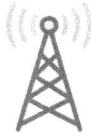

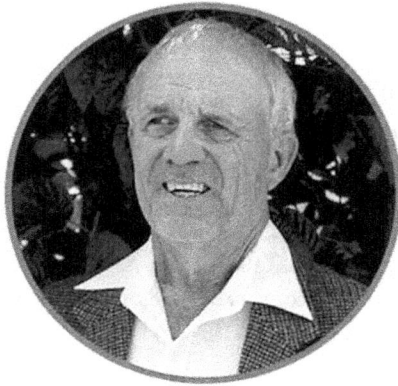

Regenerative Farmer, Geobiologist,
EMF Radiation Specialist

ABOUT THE AUTHOR: DAVID LANGE

David Lange has been an EMF Consultant since 2016. He works mainly in the rural areas of Queensland, Australia, assisting clients in identifying and mitigating EMF issues and challenges that contribute to and impact them detrimentally in their residences and workplaces.

David grew up enthusiastic about primary production, nurturing the soil, and growing nutritious food at his family property. After graduating with First Class Honours from Agricultural College, David returned to work on the family farm, where he commenced his real education. He challenged current agricultural practices by applying innovative techniques and emerging scientific research and by adopting nature's philosophy of continually looking for ways to improve oneself.

Investigating soil nutrition harnessed his passion to look further at the interconnectedness of soil and how its functioning is integral to the well-being of nature and, ultimately, human health. He learned that to create wholesome, nutrient-dense food, the vigor of the landscape and its components need to function synergistically. As David's knowledge grew, he applied what is now known as Regenerative Agriculture to balance the landscape components and improve its interconnectedness. Despite these initiatives, there was still something more. The missing link became apparent when he saw a photo of a maize crop. The plants growing near power lines were severely stunted. The invisible EMFs in the maize's environment harmed this portion of the crop's overall well-being.

David's introduction to GEOVITAL, the ability to assess, identify, and alleviate EMF's harmful impacts, was integral to restoring optimum health in a family member and understanding its detrimental implications in the broader environment. Since then, he has been using his EMF knowledge to educate and assist clients in improving their well-being. Additionally, David presents to audiences in a wide range of networks, providing EMF education, designing solutions for clients' homes and work environments, and liaising with health practitioners in the broader public.

David's passion is sharing his EMF knowledge to inform and empower others to support and improve their quality of life and the environments in which they live, work, and play.

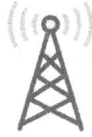

CHAPTER 3

SOURCES OF EMF - RADIO FREQUENCY RADIATION

By David Lange

Greetings and welcome to my chapter on Radio Frequency Radiation.

After reading this chapter, I trust that you will be informed to identify the sources of radio frequency radiation that may have daily impacts on you and your family. This chapter will review the sources that emit the higher frequency of EMFs. These sources have significantly increased since the early 1900s, and with technological gains since the 1990s, the times in our lives when we are exposed to them have increased dramatically. One problem has always been the need for more independent assessments to examine the long-term safety of these new devices and technologies.

In May 2011, IARC (International Agency for Research on Cancer, a part of the World Health Organization WHO), in press release #208, declared that radio frequency waves are a Group 2B possible carcinogen. It is these radio frequency waves that are emitted by mobile phones.

Radio frequencies are part of the electromagnetic spectrum below infrared. The two parts of any radio frequency are the wavelength and photons. The wavelength in this spectrum section varies from several kilometres for AM radio waves to 1mm for the microwave range. The number of waves per second, or frequency, increases as these waves decrease in length or wavelength. These frequencies are expressed in Hertz (Hz). The photons carry the energy of the radio frequency. The energy at which these radio waves are transmitted gives them range or how far they will travel.

The power potential of radio frequency is often expressed as volts (V), while the power consumed is often expressed as watts (W). The energy of one photon increases as you move higher up the electromagnetic spectrum. These photons all move at the same speed in a vacuum: the speed of light. The part of the electromagnetic spectrum we will examine in this chapter will be 100kHz to 300 GHz.

History:

The use of radio waves for communications has now been with us for over 100 years. Although they were first discovered in the 19th century, it was during World War 1 that radio waves were developed into communication systems by coupling, receiving and transmitting functions into one device. Hence, the first two-way radios were large and primarily stationary units. While the line of sight between devices was considered the limiting factor to the range between devices, it was discovered that bouncing the radio waves off the ionosphere could extend the range to over 1000 kilometres (625 miles). After the end of the war, AM radio emerged, bringing news and entertainment to the public.

The walkie-talkie, or handheld two-way radio, was the forerunner to our modern mobile phones, which was important during World War 2. This period also saw the advent of radar systems to detect enemy presence, giving the attacked a chance to defend themselves.

Radio wave technologies were developed over the next few decades, and other uses emerged. Television and radiotelephone systems began to fill our airspace with their signals. The first mobile phone systems were developed in the late 1940s; however, they only became prominent in the late 1980s when they could be made more portable and affordable. As the phone companies sold more phones, prices lowered, and more people could afford them. Paging machines also became popular in some workplaces where a person needed to be alerted, but their exact location was often changing or unknown. As mobile phone systems have developed over time, they have incorporated many new features where data rather than speech is their primary use. The latest mobile phones often come with Bluetooth and WiFi applications to exchange data in different situations.

The Internet or computer-to-computer communication has existed since the 1960s. In the 1990s, it expanded to the World Wide Web. At first, these computer-to-computer communications used a wired system; however, radio frequency emitting WiFi and hot spotting of other devices have made this more efficient and convenient.

Now that computer chips or microchips have been made much smaller and more powerful, they are used in many aspects of our daily lives. Many tools, devices, and toys use these tiny microchips to perform tasks and monitor things in our daily lives. By using radio frequencies, these microchips relay information to each other and can take these messages and information to another part of the world.

Where can you find Radio Frequency Radiation in your life?

Mobile Telephones

Mobile phone technology has now been integrated into almost every part of our lives. The expanding number of mobile phone users and the different applications the technology has incorporated into them have seen an explosion in the use of radio waves.

The mobile phone network relies on a series of phone towers across the landscape to make it work. When you make a call, your phone links with a signal to the antenna of a phone tower to transfer your conversation to the person you have called, either on another mobile phone or a landline. Each phone tower has a designated area it will cover so that when you move, your phone will automatically search for the next phone tower, which it needs to log onto. The coverage area of a phone tower needs to overlap with at least one other phone tower. To make the mobile phone system function seamlessly, it is necessary to have a series of phone towers with antennas.

Phone towers are located where they have some height to minimise physical barriers, get better coverage, and provide stronger signals. Some phone towers have been disguised as trees or palms, while in other situations, antennas have been coloured and shaped to fit in with the surrounding architecture. They are regularly attached to higher buildings, and hospitals are often used where more susceptible people are.

Antennas on Phone Towers

Generally, most cell phone towers will have two types of antennas on them. The round drums, which can be large, are for communication between phone towers. Signals between the phone towers are relatively strong, and the drums focus on one another. As the signal radiates from the drum, it spirals out and affects a larger area. This is often across populated areas, so multiple houses are being affected by these signals on their path to the next tower drum. These signals could affect your house heavily, but when you look at the landscape, you would think the burden would be much lower.

The smaller square and rectangular-shaped antennas on the phone towers receive and send signals between the mobile phone and the phone tower. Multiples of these antennas are positioned around the phone tower for more complete coverage. Each mobile phone carrier generally has its own set of phone towers. In the heavier populated areas, more phone towers are being built to handle the increase in service providers, or multiple carriers may hang their antennas on the same tower.

Mobile phone handsets have come a long way since the concept was first considered. As they have progressed, the technology used has been physically condensed in size and has increased in the capabilities and the functions it can perform. Instant and continuous data is an ever-expanding use of mobile phones in business. Social messaging via different mobile phone apps has also increased the use of mobile phones by many people.

We have progressed from analogue systems to 2G, 3G, 4G and 5G (5G = 5th generation of technology). Each generation of mobile phones uses different wavebands and coverage maps. Demand requires new networks to carry more data with quicker delivery. People's need for more data quicker is an ongoing dilemma, spiralling faster and faster.

Only some realise that network development is responding to consumer demand. In the time of 2G, we also started to use mobile phones for Skype voice calls, and our data needs increased. The mobile phone user needed 3G, and it came. 4G came when we had progressed to making video calls, and faster data transfers were required. We're now in the era of YouTube and Netflix streaming, which coincides with 5G. The more data we, as consumers, ask for, the more the industry will get ready for it. That is why 6G is already in development and expected to have pre-commercial trails from 2028, and the first commercial 6G services will be available around 2030. Unless you and many other people stop using data… we are all part of the reason our exposure to radio frequency radiation is increasing.

Since about 2019, the 5G network has rolled out worldwide. Mobile phone carriers are utilising a wide range of radio wave frequencies to give their 5G network, range of transmission, and volume of data. In Australia, 5G super towers operate 5G in the low band and mid-band, incorporating Standalone and mm beam forming. This mm beam forming is a technology where the signal to your phone is targeted like a laser beam from the tower to your phone and back again. The beams will get wider as you move away from the towers and reach over 5 metres (16 feet) wide, affecting the mobile phone user and anybody in the beam. The radio frequency radiation in the beam is much more concentrated and follows you as you move. The 100 milliwatts WHO recommended exposure level within these beams can be exceeded.

As the number of cell phone users and our demand for data increase worldwide, the amount of radio waves in the environment will also increase. We must be aware that we are driving this push for faster networks that emit more radio frequency radiation with increasingly capable technology.

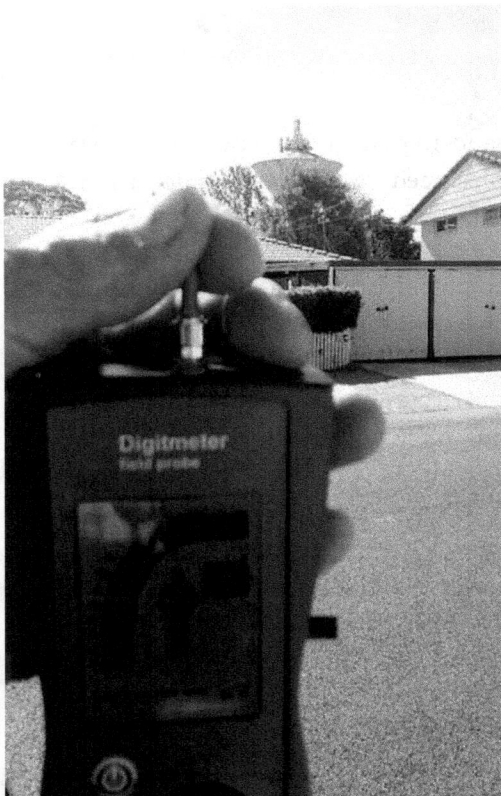

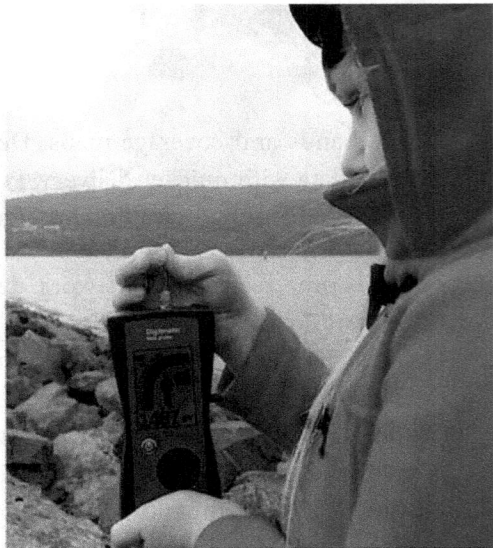

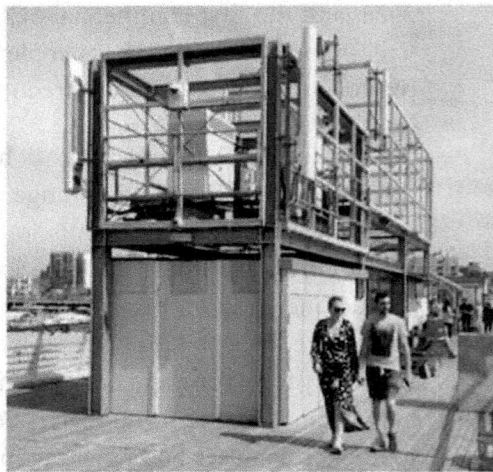

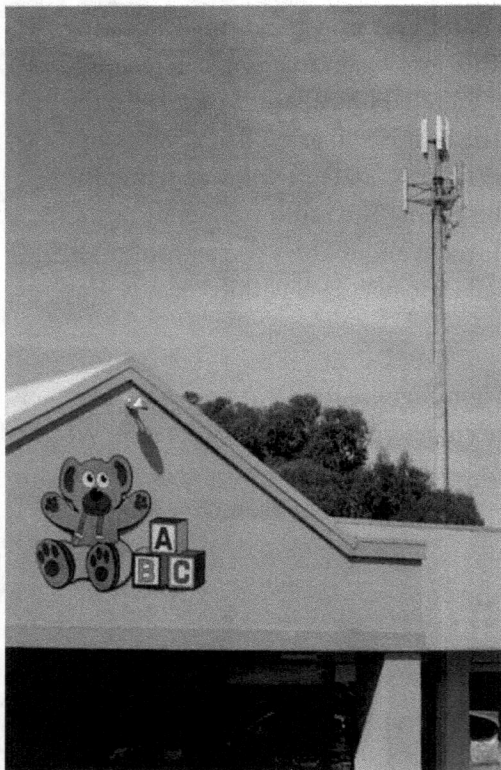

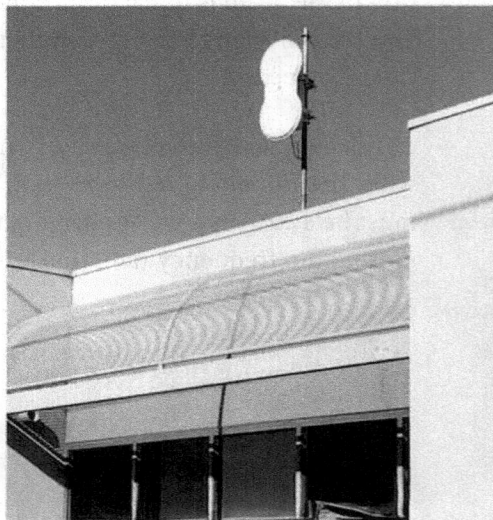

WiFi

WiFi is a short-range wireless technology that transmits data over short distances in a LAN (Local Area Network). WiFi was originally a shortened form of Wide Fidelity, but it has become known as short for Wireless Fidelity through advertising programs. WiFi became available commercially in the late 1990s and became more popular, and now virtually every mobile phone and laptop computer has it as standard. You can access the internet from your device if you are on a LAN. You can also disable this on devices.

WiFi typically operates on the 2.4GHz and 5GHz radio frequencies. Channels are allocated within these frequency bands to increase the data used within the network. The power transmission of WiFi is usually up to 100 milliwatts. When obstructions such as walls and plant life are in the way, the 2.4 GHz frequency will give a more precise signal over a longer distance than the higher 5 GHz frequency. The typical range for most WiFi networks is 10 to 30 metres (33 to 100 feet), with some expanding to 100 metres (330 feet). With a WiFi extender, it is possible to enhance the signal to further away places from the same router.

The internet is being delivered to remote villages in poorer regions using WiFi signals. By establishing a system of solar-powered nodes across the area, data and communications are brought to these people.

WiFi is used in rural areas to bring or improve mobile reception to the property. The erection of a high aerial makes a connection with a phone tower. The signal from this is beamed across your property using WiFi technology, giving better reception to your phone.

Bluetooth

Bluetooth is another short-range wireless technology that generally uses radio waves over distances up to 10 metres (33 feet). The radio waves usually have a bandwidth of 2.402 GHz to 2.48 GHz. Bluetooth's power transmission is generally limited to 2.5 milliwatts. It often exchanges data between fixed and mobile devices where cabling is restrictive or problematic. Bluetooth is most effective over smaller distances as it has fewer possible devices to manage.

Routers

The router gives you access to the internet, typically through WiFi signals. You can turn off the WiFi on many units, not all, with a simple switch. WiFi on the routers that do not have a switch can be disabled by going into the service provider's portal and disabling it. You can enjoy faster connectivity (a selling point for the kids) by using a cable connection instead. In Chapter 6, you will find out how to change to a wired connection, which is easy, and how to reduce the effects if you insist on using WiFi.

Smart Meters

Smart meters have become the preferred metering device for energy and utility providers. The meter will consist of two parts, one to read the quantity of the service being used (e.g., electricity) and the other to be a communication system that sends the data to a central receiving point.

These Smart electricity meters have the potential to produce dirty electricity, which will then circulate through your home. In some models, the data was sent back to the company through the power lines, affecting the current quality delivered to the premises. Today, this data communication happens through a mobile phone network or a low-speed wireless connection. The low-speed wireless network will link a group of houses together in the street in a Home Area Network (HAN) hub. The HAN will be mounted in the street and data will be transmitted to the energy company via a mobile phone link. This establishes a network that functions similarly to a WiFi network. This means every meter and HAN is another cell phone in or near your house, making a call at least every 30 minutes.

Location of the Meter Box / Smart Meter

The location of these Smart meters is also an issue. The meter box is often attached to the outside wall of the house, and since there are commonly more bedrooms in a home than other room types, there is a high chance it will be a bedroom wall. So, while the person is sleeping, they are exposed to this radio frequency radiation all night long. With land developments, the allotments are becoming smaller, and the house is taking up a more significant portion of the property. Being closer to your neighbour also means you will be closer to their Smart meter and exposed to their radiation.

Water and gas utility organisations also use Smart meter technology to record and read customer usage. Now, more than one meter could be producing radio frequency radiation on your property.

T98 shielding paint and Nova shielding fabric are effective in shielding your bedroom and home from the radio frequency radiation generated by these Smart meters (See Chapters 7 and 8 about mitigation).

Cordless Phone

Cordless phones have become popular in many households and businesses, giving the user the ability to be away from the base handset when taking or making a call, as well as being able to keep moving. A cordless phone works like a mobile phone but on a much smaller range and different frequencies. Much of the radiation you will be impacted by comes through the antenna, so it is essential to keep the antenna away from your body. Many base stations can transmit non-stop radio frequencies in your home with or without a call going on.

Radar

The military developed radar in the 1930s and 1940s for defence purposes. Radar uses frequency in the microwave range of the electromagnetic spectrum. A radar sends a short pulse of electromagnetic energy in a beam into space from an antenna. When this beam hits an object, it reflects a portion of this energy to the antenna. Operators determine the object's size, range, and speed from this reflected energy, e.g., an aircraft.

Depending on where you live, radar could be a cause for concern. There are studies linking radar to health risks and cancer. Airports, harbours and military bases have radar installations, which may affect many homes around them. Weather forecasting services use radar to help predict and locate storm system movements. Their location is usually in less populated areas, but they can also be in built-up areas.

While having a body assessment for radio frequency radiation done, you can, in that case, hear the radar 'coming past' at regular intervals with a sweeping

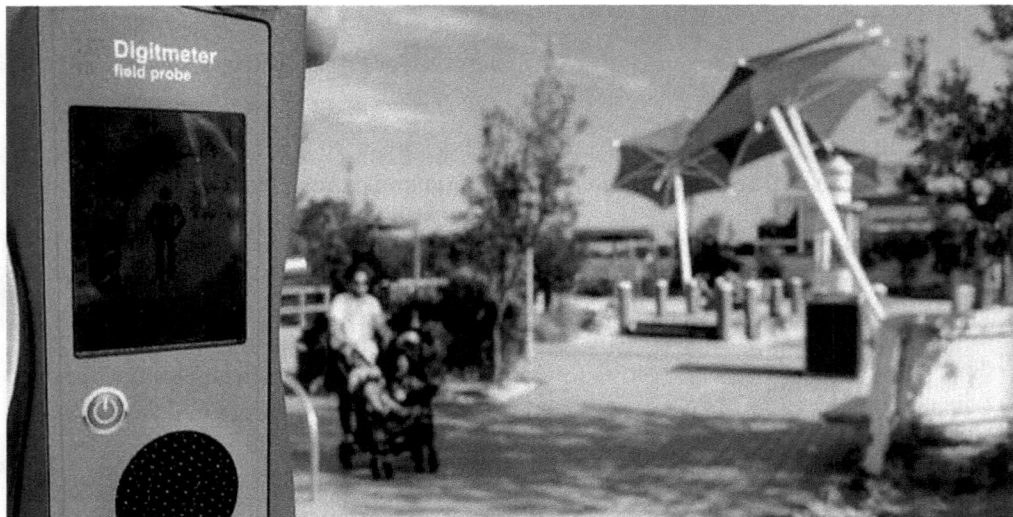
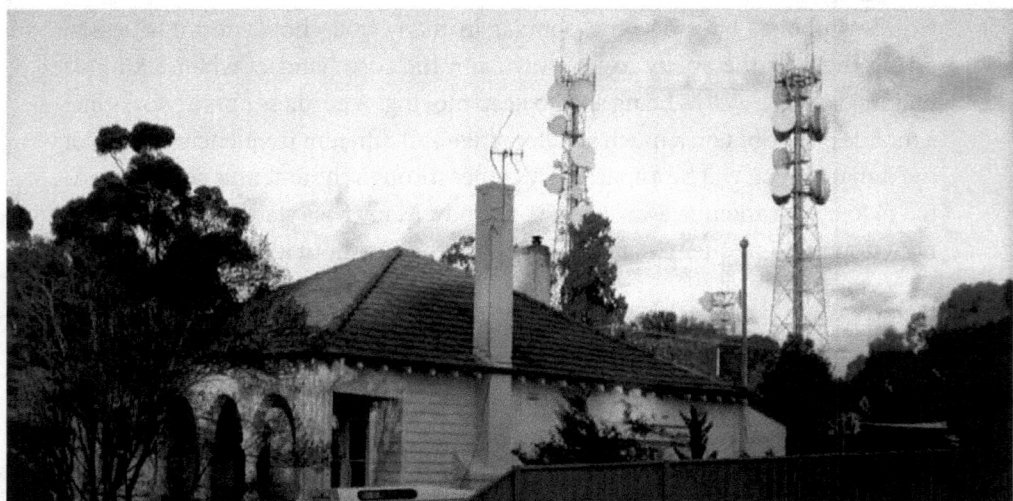
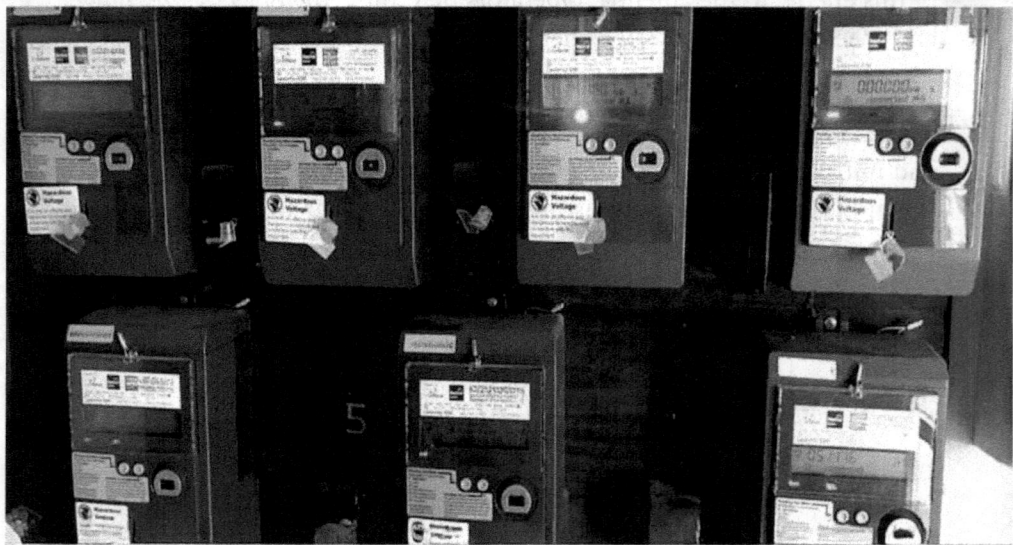

sound. A famous documentary about light, called 'Exploring The Spectrum' by Dr John Ott, which can be found on YouTube, shows aphids on the leaves of an orange tree that do a little dance (shock movement) at regular intervals. According to Dr. Ott, the aphid's dance timing correlated with the radar's rotation rate at the nearby airport, which was 14 miles away (22 Km).

Dr Ott observed this in 1974 when ongoing exposure to phone tower radiation didn't exist. It makes you wonder if the aphids still have time not to be affected. (Look up the documentary at https://youtu.be/BOUA8UAEAdY and go to the 1hr 9min mark.) T98 shielding paint and Nova shielding fabric are effective for radar radiation in the home or bedroom (See Chapters 7 and 8 about mitigation).

Phone Towers

In our experience, on average, the primary source of radio frequency radiation exposure on the human body is from phone towers. Phone towers can be large and prominent but also small, camouflaged and hidden in pillars and under utility hole covers in the street. Their radiation reaches deep into our homes, and the exposure doesn't stop and tends to increase over time with more coverage and newer networks.

Regarding your exposure, these are some things you should know: radio frequency radiation comes from the phone towers around you directly to the homes in its coverage network. What needs to be understood is that the directional transmitters (the round drums) connect the phone towers. If your home is near a phone tower or in between two phone towers, there is a high likelihood that you are 'shot in the back' by the phone tower you're not looking at. We have had health clients who worked out themselves, that they were on the centreline between two phone towers. Regular headaches were the complaints. After an assessment was completed, they put advised shielding in place, then the headaches went away.

Concrete and double brick walls can slightly reduce the amount of radio frequency radiation coming through. Unfortunately, this is much less the case for timber homes. Windows are more permeable to radio frequency radiation, so the more glass you have, in combination with them facing the

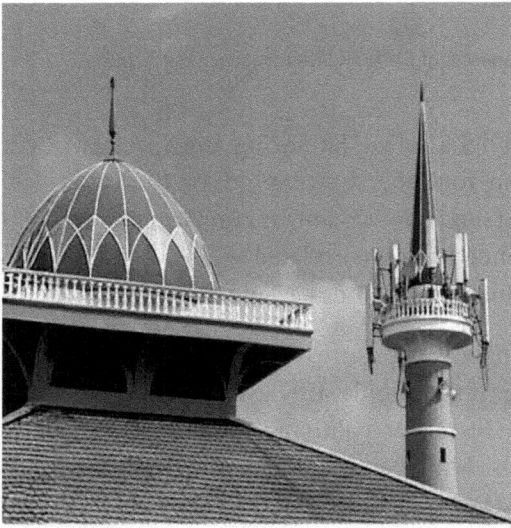
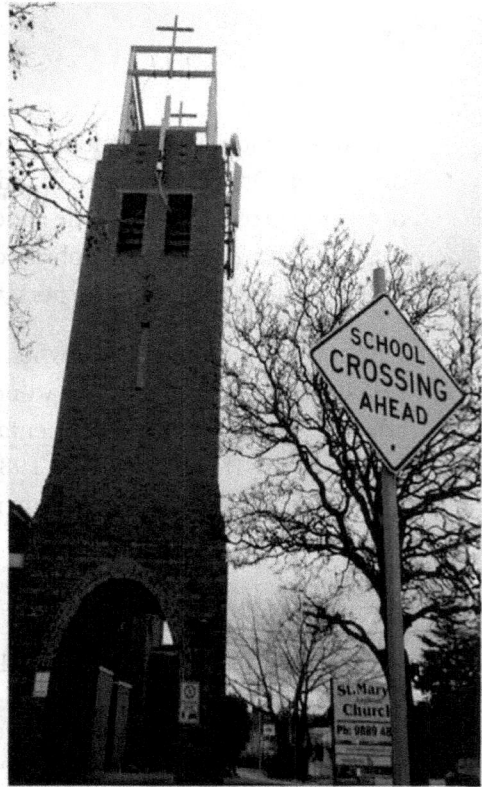
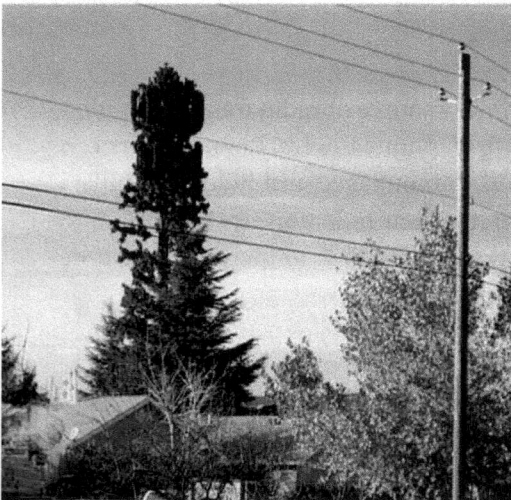
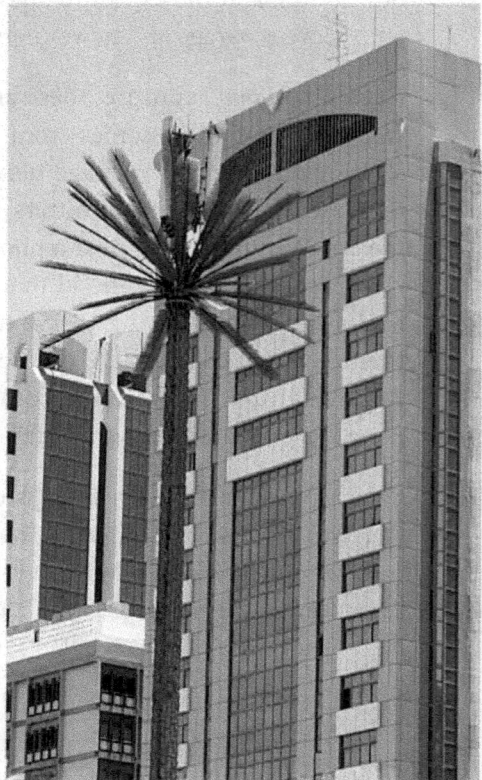
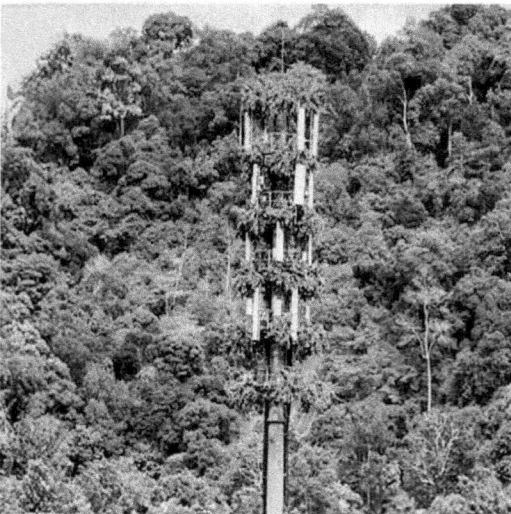

direction of phone towers, the more radio frequency radiation exposure you'll likely find coming in.

Homes with a view of the city also tend to have higher readings because in that view are many phone towers with a direct view of that home.

Other Gadgets

To identify WiFi and Bluetooth-enabled devices and appliances, you should pay attention to the marketing of these items. Check the advertising and the packaging for the WiFi and Bluetooth symbols. Gadgets, controlled by App assistant products like Amazon Alexa and Hey Google, bring radio frequency radiation into your life. The simple word 'Smart' is one of the most significant clues. It suggests that a household gadget can think for itself or is so good that it can perform menial tasks for you. We can control and monitor these gadgets when we are out by being able to link to the internet, computer, or mobile phone. They need radio frequencies to achieve this.

More devices that use wireless connections

The number of devices with WiFi and Bluetooth working in the background might surprise you.

Examples of devices with WiFi and Bluetooth capabilities in and around your home

Home Office	Kitchen
Laptops & Computer	Dishwasher & Washing machines
Internet router	Refrigerator & Deep freezer
Tablets & Mobile phones	Robotic vacuum cleaner
Printers, Keyboards and the mouse	Cooking appliances
	Cordless phone
Lounge Room	
Smart televisions	**Bed & Bathroom**
Air conditioning & Cooling fans	Heating & cooling mattress cover
Gaming devices & controllers	Baby monitors
Audio speakers	Sleep headphones
Hey Google & Amazon Alexa-controlled devices	Bathroom scales
Light & Ceiling fan controls	Speech-controlled alarm clock
Home security & Video surveillance systems	
Doorbells & Door locks	**Outdoors**
Tracking gadgets for Keys, Remotes, Wallet	Remote control garage doors & Front gates
Pet Camera	Personal Exercise Equipment
	Swimming pool filtration systems
Personal	Garden watering systems
Hearing aids	Robotic lawn mowers
Fitness monitors & Health tracking devices	Gas BBQ or Outdoor grill
Children	**Unexpected Places**
Remote control ride-on toys	Nappies with sensors
Robot pets	Baby body temperature monitor
Toothbrush	Pot plant monitors

While this is not an exhaustive list of all the potential sources of radio frequency radiation, it will give you clues about the likely sources. As new technologies are developed and marketed, these sources will expand into new, unsuspecting areas.

Now embedded in our lifestyle, radio frequency radiation exposure needs to be diligently limited and shielded against, especially focusing on the sleep areas of the home (the place our bodies rest and repair and the place we have most control) to reduce our exposure to a level that doesn't impact our health. As the effects of EMF radiation, of which radio frequency radiation is a part, are cumulative, always remember it was the last straw that broke the camel's back.

I trust that you are now more informed about radio frequency radiation and its sources.

I'm based near Dalby in Queensland, Australia. Should you need my assistance with your home, you can connect with me via the QR code.

CONNECT WITH ME

David Lange
Regenerative Farmer, Geobiologist,
EMF Radiation Specialist

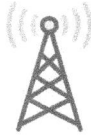

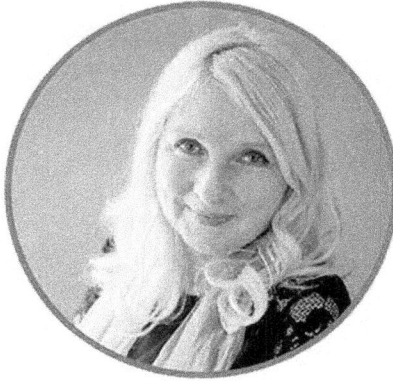

Beata Rakowski

EMF Radiation Specialist, Geobiologist,
Activist, Polyglot

ABOUT THE AUTHOR:
BEATA RAKOWSKI

Beata Rakowski is a qualified GEOVITAL EMF radiation consultant in British Columbia, Canada. She is widely involved in public consultations and advocates for awareness about the demonstrated dangers of EMF radiation and the need for safe technology. Her drive to spread awareness of EMF dangers among local governments was instrumental in stopping a cell tower proposal on Canada's West Coast.

Beata's diverse background in film and television production, extensive travel, and proficiency in multiple languages enabled her to become an accomplished translator and teacher. Later, she transitioned into social work, positively empowering many individuals who faced difficult times.

Experiencing health problems caused by excessive electrical field and wireless radiation exposure at her home, she realized how devastating this can be on the human body. After a home assessment with an EMF consultant, Beata found her way to the GEOVITAL Academy for Radiation Protection and Geobiology.

She strongly desired to learn all she could about holistic solutions to protect herself and others. Through professional training and ongoing specialization, she obtained specific knowledge to deal with EMF radiation in a manner that suits a long-term holistic approach to a healthy life. As a result, she restored her health, and is well-qualified to assist others. Her experience perfectly illustrates how an open mind and initiative may lead to positive changes and opportunities.

During home assessments, Beata uses professional instruments to accurately assess the body for radiation frequency exposure and to reliably identify zones where the body may be under stress.

She advises her clients on how to successfully mitigate EMF radiation in their homes, with the aim of enabling the body to repair itself and restore well-being.

For your Home Assessment, please reach out to Beata at Radiation Free Life

www.radiationfreelife.com

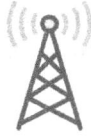

CHAPTER 4

HOW TO USE AN AMATEUR EMF METER

By Beata Rakowski

Welcome to my chapter on using an EMF meter, and congratulations on taking steps towards creating a healthier and safer home environment. I have seen the impacts of EMF radiation exposure firsthand and love helping people through proper home assessments. It's my pleasure to share some essential insights regarding purchasing and using a quality EMF meter.

This chapter will focus on amateur meters and their practical application as instruments for assessing radiation exposures around us. You will learn the purpose and features of an EMF meter, how to select one, recommended exposure levels, and how to find problem sources inside and outside the home.

In today's technology-saturated world, owning an EMF meter is as essential as your car's headlights when driving through the night to guide you safely home, since these instruments make the invisible dangers visible.

NOTE: EMF radiation exposure problems are not insurmountable, and there are solutions. While I would urge anyone to purchase a good amateur EMF meter, addressing concerns in your home should be done through a professional who assesses the home and your body's exposure to EMF's. They should be trained in EMF mitigation, be familiar with your home situation, able to devise a sound mitigation approach based on experience, and be available to support you to turn your home into a healthy environment.

What is important when choosing EMF meters?

EMF meters are multi-functional devices designed to evaluate various forms of non-ionizing radiation found in our environment, including homes. If you have not purchased an amateur EMF meter already, this chapter contains valuable information. EMF meters can range in price from a modest price to thousands of dollars. However, as with most products, the price is usually indicative of the quality. The question is, how do you select a reliable EMF meter?

You want an EMF meter that can test for the three most common radiation types:

- Magnetic Fields (MF)
- Electric Fields (EF)
- Radiofrequency Radiation (RF)

Magnetic Fields (MF)

For magnetic fields, I am of the opinion that you need a quality tool with a 3-axis sensor in the meter.

Magnetic fields sort of spin in a direction, a bit like a spinning plate, if that analogy helps you. The single-axis meter **does not give you all the information** in one reading as you have to turn it in different directions, record the readings, followed by a mathematical calculation. If this process is not observed, you may think there is low exposure, when in fact, it is high.

A 3-axis meter does not require to be turned in several directions nor require calculations. It should read reasonably accurate, no matter how it is orientated.

Electric Fields (EF)

Electric fields are a common radiation type found in nearly all homes and bedrooms. Most sleeping areas have exposure levels that are way higher than our health-focused industry recommends. As a consultant, I consider it a necessity to own a reasonably sensitive meter to assess such electric fields in the home. Because our bodies are electrically conductive, taking readings of a person's body, not the air, would be ideal. Most people are completely unaware of the presence of electric fields they are exposed to on a daily basis, especially in their bedrooms, and the adverse impacts this has on their bodies.

Radiofrequency Radiation (RF)

Radiofrequency radiation is emitted by phone towers, radar, Wi-Fi, smart meters, cordless phones, and other wireless technologies. Generally, the higher the range the meter can assess (3Ghz, 4Ghz, 5Ghz, 6Ghz, etc.), the better it is. It's important to note that the frequency range advertised on the box may not always be reliable, and some meters may under-read compared to professional or quality amateur meters.

Secondary Features

The most crucial aspect of a meter is the accuracy of the information it provides. While it is nice to have additional features, they are of little use if the meter is not precise, sufficiently sensitive and dependable.

Secondary features that can be valuable for a good EMF meter:

- Peak Hold, handy for seeing the highest value, even if it was just for a few seconds

- The ability to easily select what radiation type you want to investigate

- A history graph to show you what happened a few minutes ago

- Back lighting so you can use it without a flashlight in low light conditions

- Audible warning sounds based on exposure levels

- Logging ability to record exposure levels over a longer period for reviewing

- Sturdy construction

How much should you pay?

Since you will make important decisions with this meter you are about to purchase, I consider it justified to invest in a quality instrument.

The Trifield TF2 was recommended to a large audience of attending medical professionals at the International EMF Medical Conference 2021. I still use my TF2 (my first meter) at community events to raise awareness about EMF exposure. When considering purchasing an EMF meter, you might like to check the price of the TF2, as it will give you a benchmark for the price and performance of a quality EMF meter. Given its features and durability, I feel the Trifield TF2 is a well-priced instrument.

Features of the Trifield TF2 meter:

While there are various amateur meters on the market, the Trifield TF2 stands out due to its excellent display, easy operation, and robust casing. Some other features are:

- AC magnetic 3-axis sensor, allowing for more accurate readings regardless of meter orientation

- Audio Indicator: (you can activate or deactivate) which emits sounds useful in pinpointing EMF sources

- Peak Hold value displayed, showing the highest exposure levels in the last few seconds

- Operates for more than 20 hours on a 9V battery

If you need more confidence, encouragement, and example videos beyond this chapter, follow the QR code at the end of my chapter; it will take you to a link where you can purchase a worthwhile online course for the TF2 with a discount.

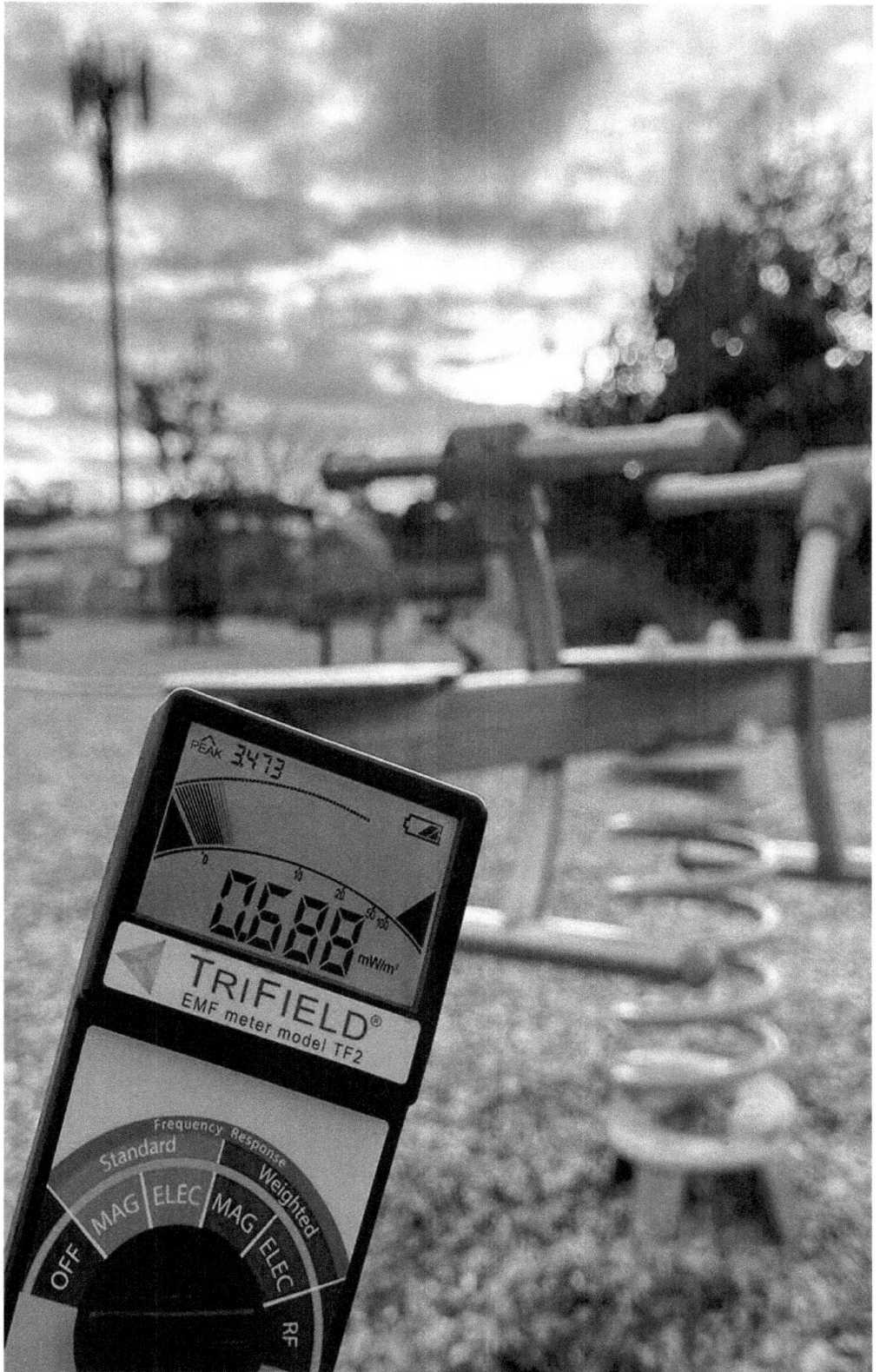

Recommended guidelines levels

It is crucial to identify the safety values and take action accordingly.

Air assessing meters tend to show radio frequency radiation in microwatts per square meter ($\mu W/m^2$) or milliwatts per square meter (mW/m^2).

Magnetic fields are usually measured in milligauss (mG) or nanotesla (nT), while electric fields are measured in volts per meter (V/m).

This table will help you understand exposure values, which you can use to set safe limits for your family. The reading on your EMF meter should ideally be as low as possible.

EMF Guidelines

	Slight Concern	Severe Concern	Extreme Concern
RF in milliwatts	0.0001-0.01 mW/m²	0.01-1 mW/m²	>1 mW/m²
RF in microwatts	0.1-10 µW/m²	10-1000 µW/m²	>1000 µW/m²
Magnetic fields in mG	0.3-1 mG	1-3 mG	>3 mG
Magnetic fields in nT	30-100 nT	100-300 nT	>300 nT
Electric field **not holding** meter	0.3-1.5 V/m	1.5-10 V/m	>10 V/m
Electric field **holding** meter	1 – 5 V/m	5-50 V/m	>50 V/m

In bedrooms, for long term, it's important to address any concerns that exceed two-thirds of the slight concern range, as they should be undisturbed 'sanctuaries' where we regenerate during sleep.

For those with microwave sickness, aka **Electromagnetic-Hypersensitivity (EHS)**, the entire range of slight concerns may also warrant improvement. Try to reduce the levels as low as possible.

TIP: For convenience, you might like to tape the most relevant information, such as 'Slight Concern' values, to the back of your meter.

For anyone who is highly sensitive to EMFs, close or ideally less than these values would be desirable:

RF in milliwatts	0.0001 mW/m²
RF in microwatts	0.1 µW/m²
Magnetic fields in mG	0.3 mG
Magnetic fields in nT	30 nT
Electric field **not holding** meter	0.3 V/m
Electric field **holding** meter	1 V/m

NOTE: Government guidelines for exposure have been set significantly higher than these guidelines. Learn about EMF radiation research in Chapter 1.

Magnetic fields cannot be effectively or economically shielded against.

For EMF mitigation and shielding solutions, refer to Chapters 7 and 8.

Holding your EMF meter correctly

The best practice is to get used to hold the lower half of the meter and not obstruct the upper half with your hand since that's where the sensors for electric fields and radio frequencies are located. Hold the meter away from you to avoid your body creating a barrier and thus reducing RF exposure readings from behind you, which would result in lower, inaccurate readings.

Because electric fields are attracted to the body, the readings in a home are typically higher when holding the meter than when placed on a surface. If you use the reference values provided for electric fields when not holding

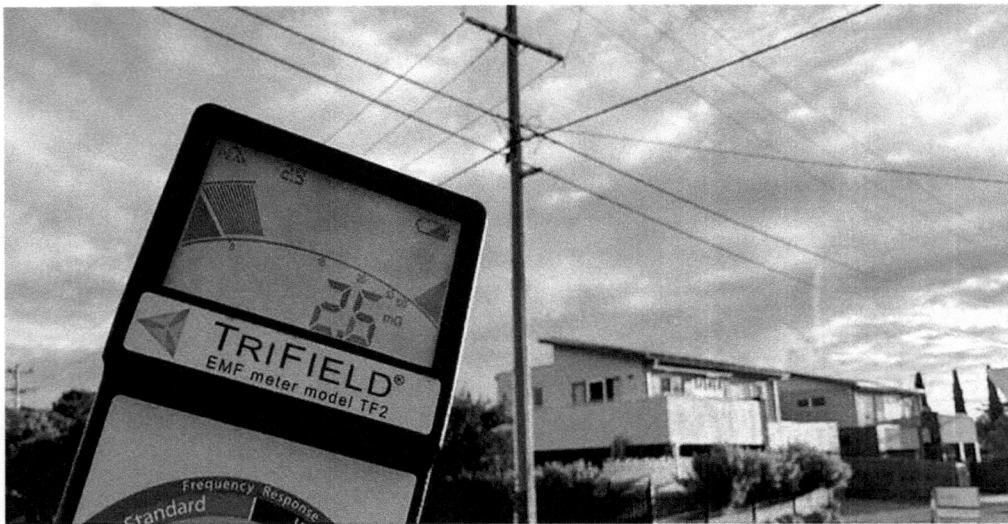

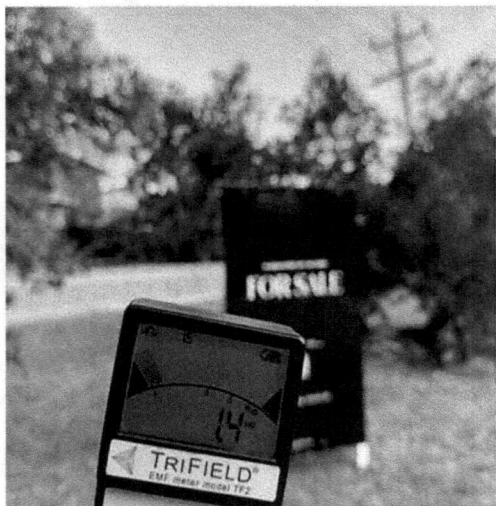

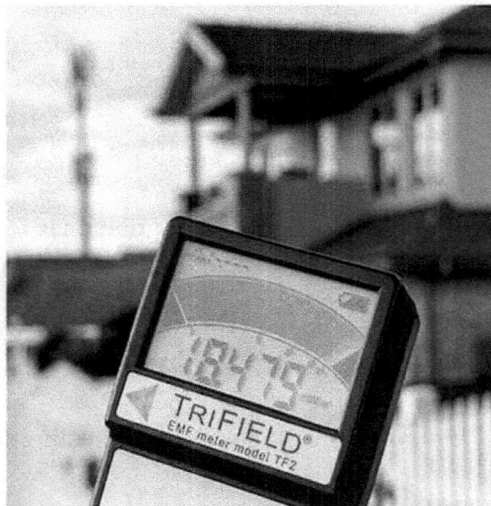

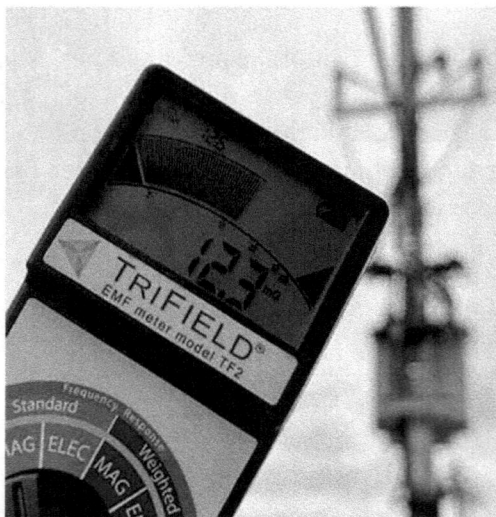

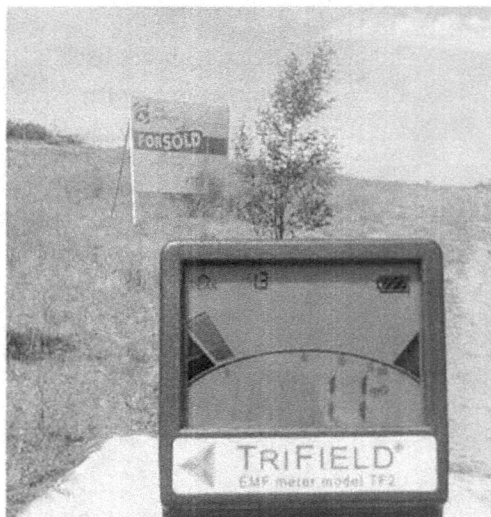

the meter, place it on a surface and step away from it as far as you can so that you can still read the display. Lowering your body to make yourself 'smaller' (by kneeling) may also be a good idea.

For electric fields it's important to use the reference values provided for 'when holding', or 'not holding' the meter. You can try moving the meter around as you stand in one place or lay on a bed to see which meter position gives you the highest reading. It is worth noting that elevated readings will likely require improvements. Remember that professional meters often indicate that the problem is more urgent.

When checking magnetic fields, avoid rapidly swinging it around and keep the meter in the same orientation. In this scenario, it is important to move the meter slowly to prevent the numbers from jumping.

Readings on screen

Your meter might display **average** and **peak** (highest) values, like the TF2 where the large number on display indicates AVERAGE, while the small PEAK number remains briefly on the screen before coming back down. When considering potential risk to the body, the highest peak readings indicate higher magnetic intensity which is problematic in the long term. Knowing that sudden movements with the meter can cause false readings, always wait a few seconds for the numbers to settle.

Using your meter on a building lot or outside an existing home

If you plan to build a home and would like to assess the property for EMFs before purchase or know the safest place to build on a property you might already own, use your meter to check for magnetic fields. For an existing home, the garden area around it can be investigated using the same method.

Set the instrument to 'Standard-MAG' (magnetic) and start to investigate the magnetic fields of the overhead or underground local distribution lines (power lines) and possible transformers at the property line near the street. What is present on the street may explain what is found on the property. You will notice that the strength of the magnetic field increases as you move closer to the source.

Walk around the perimeter, while holding the meter towards the ground in case cables or other sources are hidden underground. Corner properties usually have stronger electromagnetic fields if both streets have power lines running alongside the building lot.

Typically, you will notice reductions in magnetic fields the further you walk away from the street. If there is a street power line also at the back of the property, readings may start to increase again as you approach the power lines at the rear. Note where you have the lowest readings.

On a larger property, repeat the same by walking and assessing closer to the existing house or where the home might be built. For insights about Radiation-Free Building, please refer to Chapter 12.

Assess electric fields by setting the meter for 'Standard-ELEC' (electric) and repeating the investigation along the property line, holding the meter well before you.

For radio frequency (RF setting), take spot readings on various areas of the land. Hold the meter with your outstretched arm at eye level, or even a little higher, as your body may shield RF if it's coming from behind you. You don't need to see phone towers to have levels we would deem excessive. If the property is near a cell tower, the RF readings will likely be very high and may max out your meter.

NOTE: During this procedure, an active cell phone in your pocket or wearing a 'smart' watch will likely increase your readings as you carry the source of the radiation with you. This also applies for any person near you carrying a wireless device. I recommend leaving wireless devices in your car or further away from you, so they don't interfere with the readings of your instrument.

Using your EMF meter in the home

Let's investigate your home.

Common sources of magnetic fields are: street power lines, transformers, solar panels, inverters, and wiring errors. Electric fields emanate from electrical wiring, including those hidden inside the walls. Radiofrequency radiation are emitted by: cell towers, 'smart' meters, cordless phones, Wi-Fi, tablets, laptops, baby monitors, 'smart' watches, just to name a few. All of these radiation sources impact our well-being.

For more information on sources of magnetic, electric, and RF radiation, see Chapters 2 and 3.

IMPORTANT: While we find EMF radiation in many parts of the home, it is easy for some people to start worrying, which is not always warranted, provided they **do not** spend long periods of time in those areas. The human body rests and restores predominantly during sleep, a key regenerative time that makes the bedrooms the most important areas to reduce the effects of radiation.

Electric, Magnetic and Radio Frequency Fields

Daytime Areas – Magnetic Fields

Magnetic fields from outside can reach into the home. If the levels of magnetic fields outside your front door are high, don't expect low readings on the other side of the door. In the long term, chronic high exposure can affect your health. This is why it is so important to ensure that magnetic fields in your bedroom are at acceptable levels for a good, restorative sleep. If the exposure in your bedroom is high, it is recommended to educate yourself on the available research and its conflict with government guidelines. You can then decide whether to stay long-term or consider moving to another location.

Look for magnetic fields in areas where you spend a lot of time. Take readings throughout the living room, dining room, kitchen, and office: along/over the sofa, around the dining/kitchen table and your office chair/desk.

Household appliances can generate magnetic fields, which may cause concern for some people. However, it's important to note that the strength of magnetic fields decreases rapidly as you move away from the source. If you are frequently in a space with a magnetic field, try to turn off or remove the source, or increase the distance between you and the source. Therefore, if appliances are located away from the areas where you spend most of your time, then exposure to the magnetic fields is likely minimal and of lesser concern.

Make sure to switch on everything at home to create a 'worst-case scenario': turn on the lights, heating, cooling, etc., as it will show if any of these produce magnetic fields and affect the areas where you spend a lot of time. If these sources are off during your assessment, you will not uncover where these strong magnetic fields are coming from.

Move your meter occasionally to the floor and the ceiling. In areas where wiring or something else produces a field, you will see your instrument readings increase accordingly.

Should you detect an area with a higher magnetic field inside the home than on the outside, and solar panels and inverters have been ruled out (they don't do anything at night), the radiation most likely originates from problems within the home's electrical system. Refer to Chapter 9 for wiring errors and stray currents.

Daytime Areas – Electric Fields

Electrical wires inside the walls, extension cords, plug-in lamps, and appliances emit electric fields in the air. Even though your instrument is not designed to investigate body voltage, you can still assess the presence of these electrical fields around you. To do so, set your meter to 'Standard-ELEC'. Place the meter in areas to investigate and step back to read the display. Alternatively, hold the meter in your hand. The latter will give you a higher reading as the body attracts electric fields, which becomes part of the readings. To interpret exposure levels, refer to the recommended guidelines for electric fields 'when holding the meter'.

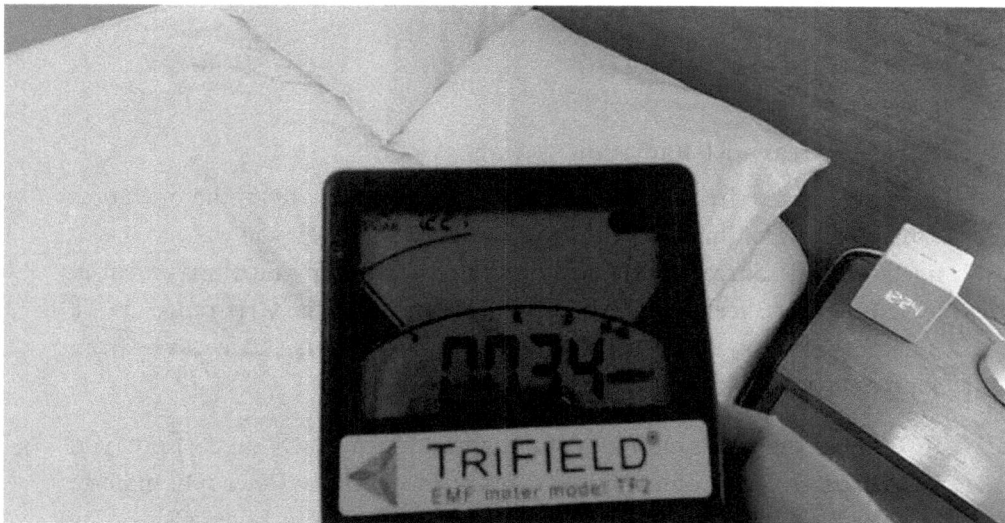

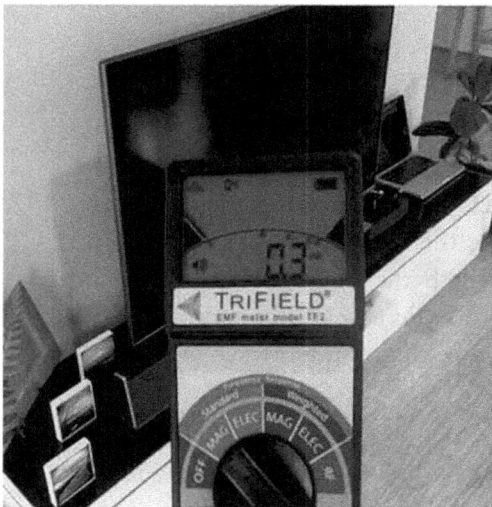

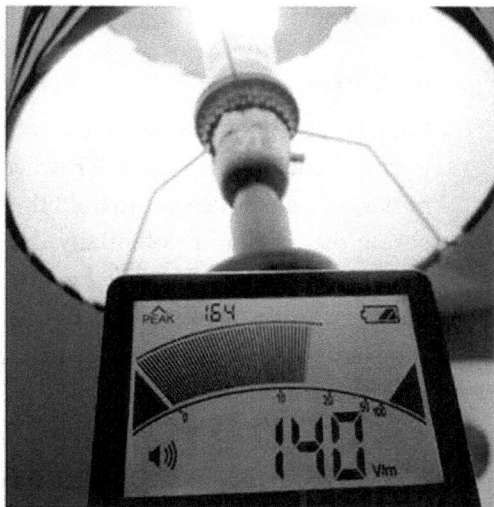

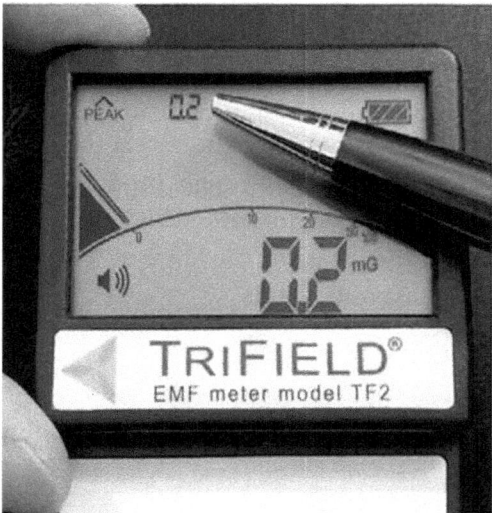

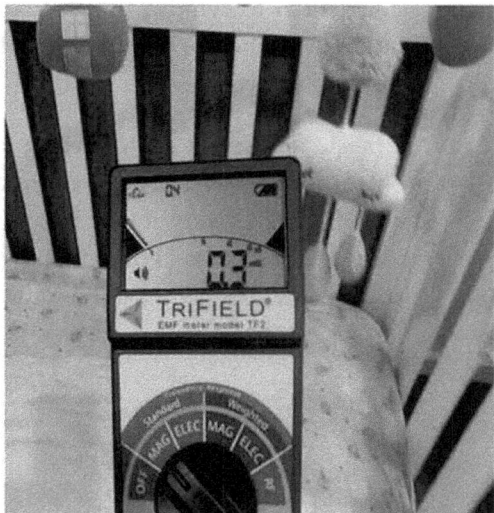

Daytime Areas – RF Radiation

To assess radio frequency radiation, remember to hold the meter as explained in 'Holding your EMF meter correctly'. When you want to investigate known sources of RF, face the source, but keep your instrument at least 1 meter / 3 feet away if there are frequencies in the GHz range (WiFi, Bluetooth, microwave oven, baby monitor) and 3 meters / 10 feet away from sources in the MHz range (amateur radio).

If you hold the meter close to your chest and turn slowly on the spot, you may discover that at one point your readings are lower. This could indicate that the biggest source of RF is now behind you as your body is shielding the meter.

RF Microwave Test

First, place a cup of water in the microwave oven, as you are not supposed to run it empty. Turn the microwave oven on and take a reading of the RF radiation. Make sure not to hold the meter too close, as it could cause inaccurate readings and potentially damage the instrument. Stand 1 meter/3 feet away and slowly walk backward with the meter between you and the microwave oven. Move away as far as you can and be prepared to be shocked about the distance at which your 'closed' microwave oven is still affecting you!

EMF radiation assessment of bedrooms

It is essential to remove the electrosmog burden from bedrooms as they should always be the priority since this is where our body is supposed to repair and rejuvenate.

Magnetic fields: just as in daytime areas, turn everything on to reveal the problem sources. While you want to discover if your lighting might produce strong magnetic fields, it is of lesser concern, as we do not sleep with lights on. The sleeping area is the most important, and assessing the levels at the corners of the bed gives a good indication of exposure levels.

Radio alarm clocks are traditionally linked to frequent headaches due to transformers found inside. The same goes for bedside touch-sensitive lamps. Water beds and electric blankets are a very poor idea, as the magnetic fields (MF) they produce are typically high when they are 'heating'. Also, motorized bed frames can produce magnetic fields during operation (some do all the time).

Electrical fields: the same procedure of assessing the bed corners for magnetic fields can be applied to detect electrical fields with the instrument setting on 'electrical fields' but this time with bedroom lights off. This will give you an idea of night time exposure to electrical fields while sleeping. Wiring inside the walls, bedside lamps, sleep apnea machines, electric clocks, and other electrical appliances, emit strong electric fields near the sleeper as long as they remain plugged into the electrical outlet. To assess electric fields, place the meter in different locations, such as behind the pillows and on the bedside table. A professional body assessment would likely indicate that the problem is more urgent.

Radio Frequency: take spot readings while standing (instrument in front) or lying on the bed, holding the meter a little away from you in different positions. It is important to understand that RF exposure can vary greatly during different times of day or night.

Final thoughts

In this chapter, my aim was to provide you with the necessary knowledge and confidence to use and interpret an EMF meter. We have covered various aspects such as what to consider when purchasing one, important values to look for, and its usage in different areas both inside and outside of your home.

Using an EMF meter is an eye-opening experience, and I hope you will not only be amazed and rightly concerned but also take action to ask for guidance on how to improve your situation. An amateur EMF meter is a good tool to own. Still, it is no substitute for a professional home assessment with meters that can assess the body for electric and RF radiation. You are a big antenna, after all. Having someone on-site who, together with you, investigates and formulates a mitigation strategy is a great start to improving your home and sleeping environments.

To gain more knowledge, confidence, and encouragement beyond this chapter, or to connect with me, follow the QR code; alternatively, reach me at www.radiationfreelife.com

I offer short, free strategy calls and, of course, EMF home assessments.

Good luck on your journey!

CONNECT WITH ME

Beata Rakowski
EMF Radiation Specialist, Geobiologist, Activist, Polyglot

https://www.radiationfreelife.com

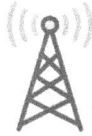

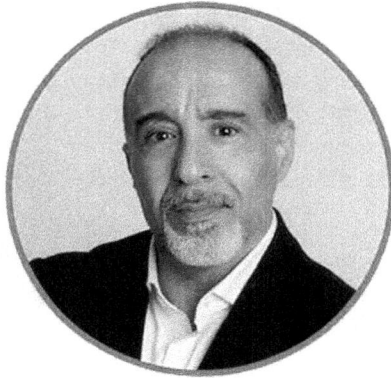

Samir Derrar
EMF Radiation Specialist, Coach

ABOUT THE AUTHOR: SAMIR DERRAR

Over the course of 22 years, UK-based Samir Derrar has built a successful career in the telecom industry. His diverse experience includes roles in RF technical support, sales and business development, and procurement of state-of-the-art electronic components for sectors such as Mobile Communication, Internet of Things (IoT), Automotive, and Satellite Communication. Samir's experience in these high-tech industries positions him as an excellent EMF consultant, offering valuable insights into the rapidly evolving wireless-connected world.

In 2016, Samir developed health issues that manifested in prolonged ringing in the ears, overwhelming fatigue, brain fog, and sleeplessness. Initially, his symptoms were dismissed, attributed to excessive business travel and work-related pressure. It was later discovered that his prolonged exposure to EMF was severely impacting his health.

Committed to reclaiming his well-being and improving the quality of his life, Samir embarked on an extensive research journey to learn about EMF – including its potential effects on health and how to deal with it safely. Within a short period, he successfully shielded his home and office, creating a radiation-free sanctuary.

Witnessing the benefits of reducing EMF exposure in his home, Samir pursued an extensive programme with Geovital International and practical training in Austria to become a professional EMF consultant. Samir then developed a keen interest in vibrational sciences that deal with hidden subtle energies – particularly Shape Therapy and BioGeometry™.

Now, Samir conducts EMF surveys across the UK and Europe. He also works with several health practitioners, including a leading holistic medical centre in London, to help their clients mitigate excessive exposure to radiation in their homes. Samir takes a practical and pragmatic approach to EMF mitigation, reassuring clients that they can reduce radiation in their homes without sacrificing the benefits and conveniences of modern technology.

In this book, Samir provides a comprehensive guide to understanding what constitutes a professional EMF home assessment and what to expect from someone offering this service. He further invites you to contact him for any queries regarding EMF and how to make your home safer and healthier for you and your family.

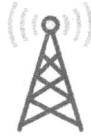

CHAPTER 5

THE PROFESSIONAL EMF HOME ASSESSMENT

By Samir Derrar

I'm thrilled that you're reading this chapter. I'm confident you will gain invaluable insights into selecting an EMF consultant to assist you and explain in more detail how to assess the various types of radiation within your home from a holistic and professional angle.

Perhaps you're reading this chapter because you're simply curious about EMF, or maybe you're experiencing health issues that have prompted you to explore their underlying causes. Perhaps you were even given a tip by a close friend that you might be electromagnetic hypersensitive and that high levels of radiation – and prolonged exposure to it – could be the root cause of your symptoms. You might have recently consulted with a holistic doctor who identified electrosmog as a factor in your diagnosis and suggested that your home or office be inspected immediately for radiation.

Upon encountering this unfamiliar term, perhaps you researched the topic and are now considering hiring a professional to conduct an EMF survey. However, before proceeding, you must determine the criteria for selecting a consultant, the specific types of radiation they should assess inside your home, and the appropriate testing equipment they should utilise.

Choosing an EMF consultant

If you're considering hiring a professional consultant for this task, it's crucial to ensure they are the most suitable choice for your needs. Generally, starting with a phone call to enquire about their offerings is a solid first step. Here are some key criteria they should meet before you proceed with engaging their services. Just be careful not to put words in their mouth regarding what you're looking for. Ask these questions and listen to what they say:

1 - How is the assessment conducted?

Regarding the home you already live in, will they run around your home on their own and give you the findings when they're finished? Every author in this book will conduct the assessment WITH the families. You will investigate together, during which you are welcome to do most of the investigating yourself, using the meters under our close supervision and guidance. We find that only then will people truly understand what is going on and will consequently learn so much more from the process. They can confidently reflect on the experience and take action to improve their situation instead of being overwhelmed by a downpour of information they don't understand and can't relate to.

2 - What radiation types do you investigate?

a. They should tell you that they investigate at least electric fields, radio frequency radiation, AND magnetic fields. Magnetic fields from outside are often unfixable and would typically stop a family from investing more in improving their space. We see this regularly: entire homes are shielded with inferior products that perform poorly, and magnetic fields are left in place because they were never investigated. The family finds no improvement and sells the house after having made an avoidable investment.

b. They must possess appropriate professional testing equipment capable of providing insights into the amount of radiation (electric and RF) absorbed by the body rather than solely focusing on air measurements. This is quite specialised, so you don't have to ask if they assess the body for RF radiation; if they have such instrumentation, they will be very keen to tell you, as it makes so much more sense than simply assessing the air. It is about the body, after all.

3 - How long will an assessment take?

I am rarely out of a home in under 2.5 hours. If they tell you their assessment takes an hour, consider what they're not doing.

4 - What do you feel is the most urgent place to assess to be safe in a home?

There is only one answer here, in my opinion. The body rests, rejuvenates, and repairs primarily during sleep. The bedroom is always the highest priority as the time spent there is key regenerative time. If you don't receive this answer, you're dealing with someone who has no idea how the body works and who clearly has no background or understanding of a holistic approach to this subject.

5 - What sort of solutions do you recommend to deal with EMF radiation when it is deemed too high?

In this scenario, what you're seeking is assurance that they provide verifiable solutions. This entails ensuring that the shielding solutions they propose to implement, along with the meters used to detect high levels of exposure, will confirm a significant reduction in exposure levels when mitigation is complete. The best way forward is to properly remove exposure to EMF and install carefully designed solutions tailored for long-term suitability, thereby creating a healthy space.

6 - What happens when things need to be fixed in the home?

An EMF consultant should be committed to follow-up and should offer guidance on selecting the most suitable shielding solutions, as well as demonstrating the sought-after positive results. More importantly, your consultant should be available for guidance during the mitigation projects you might embark on. Suppose they point you to another company to make your purchases and are unavailable for you or your tradespeople to speak to. In that case, you'll be left uncertain, doubting if things were implemented correctly. Don't get me wrong; you can easily manage mitigation in most cases, but you will no doubt have many questions. Your consultant must be readily available and supportive, even just on video calls.

In addition, these observations can be helpful:

- Their website should be content-rich, informative, and reflective of their expertise and depth of knowledge in the field. (Watch out for content created by AI, which means very little.)

- Their website should feature authentic, positive reviews that align with your EMF concerns. If in doubt, request a reference.

I trust this list of questions has given you greater confidence in approaching an EMF consultant in your area. Feel free to connect with me and request a recommendation if you'd like. Let us know your country, state, and city/town, and we'll search within our network to find someone who can assist you.

More considerations

To ensure you engage a good EMF consultant, it's essential to understand the various types of radiation, the necessary meters for testing them, and their functionalities.

While low-cost LED flashing meters might suffice for non-professionals, EMF consultants require precise and sophisticated instruments with particular specifications to ensure that a clear assessment of the situation can be made. For example, assessing radiation levels in the air differs from gauging the amount of radiation your body absorbs.

Participation in an assessment

When conducting our EMF home assessments, I encourage the client to participate in as much of the survey as possible. During this two- to three-hour home assessment, clients will learn many handy tips on how to improve their environment, particularly focusing on critical factors within the bedroom. If you have a partner, I believe it is crucial they are also present, as this will ensure understanding and easy discussion between you about any observations and recommendations made during the assessment.

Meters and testing equipment

In my view, assessing EMF in your home requires the use of two distinct types of professional and essential EMF testing equipment. The first type investigates air density, indicating radiation levels in specific areas, while the other investigates body voltage to assess how much of that radiation is absorbed by your body. Both probes capture readings of low-frequency radiation, referred to as electric fields, and radio frequency radiation (RF), also referred to as high-frequency or sometimes microwaves. Alongside the previously mentioned instrumentation, a Gauss meter is another essential instrument necessary for investigating magnetic fields. Lastly, a Dirty Electricity Meter – which assesses high spurious content on your household electricity lines – is also part of my kit.

For further insights into the distinction between amateur and professional investigation methods, please refer to Chapter 4.

Now that we've covered the types of meters necessary for a thorough and proper survey, let's explore the various forms of radiation commonly encountered in every household – and their implications.

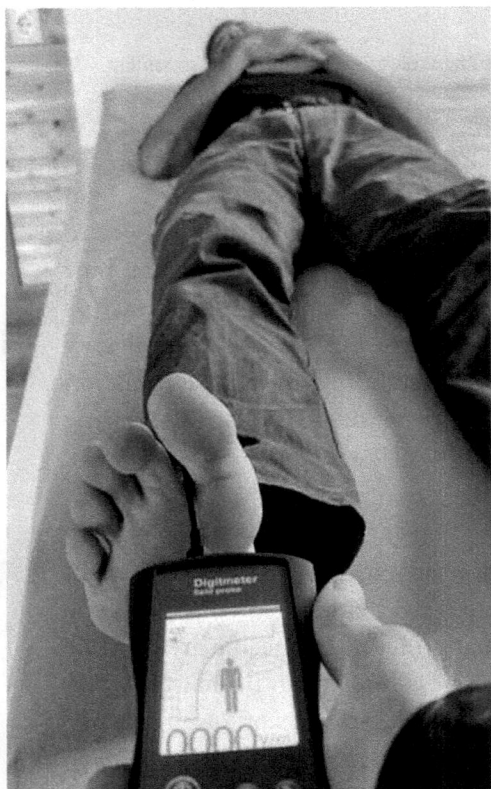
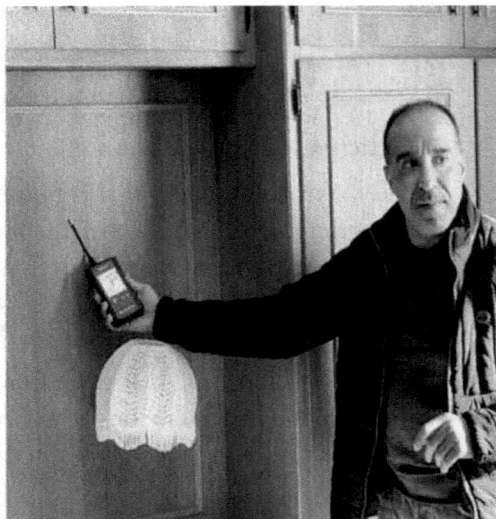
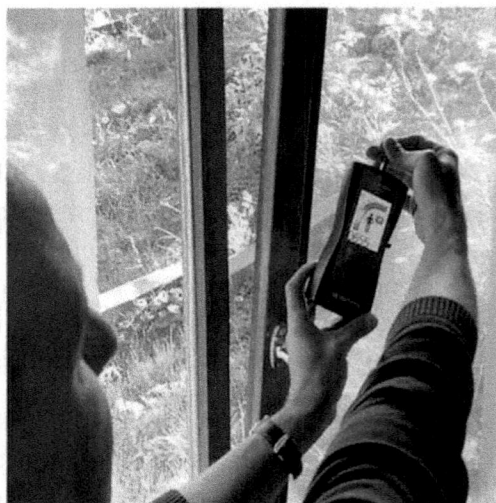
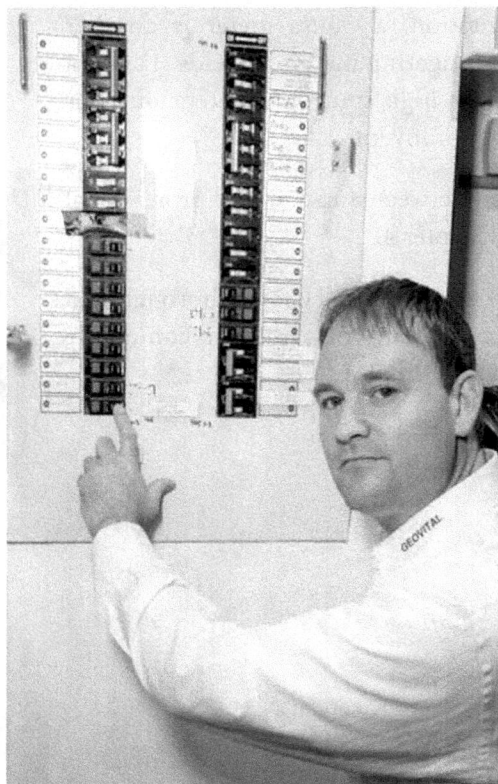
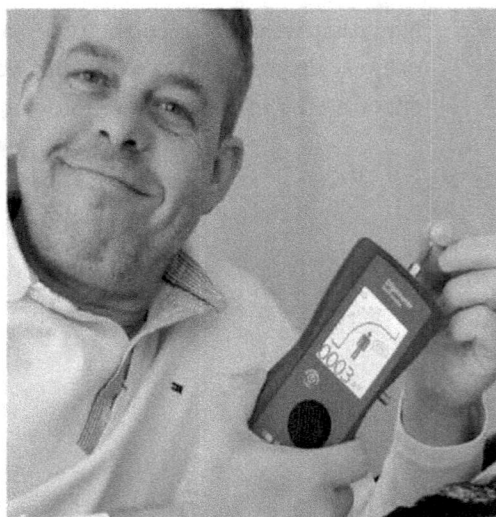

Types of EMF

EMF stands for 'electromagnetic field,' a term often used to encompass all types of low-level non-ionising radiation. Other terms used interchangeably with EMF include EMR (electromagnetic radiation), electronic pollution, and electrosmog. These come in various forms:

1. Electric Fields

These types of radiation derive from live electrical household wiring – electrical wiring that has voltage on it.

Electric fields typically extend up to 6 feet (2 metres) from their source or even farther. The strength and intensity of electric fields vary based on the voltage level of the wiring and the number of sources producing them. Unless shielded, all wiring emits this radiation, and electric fields persist on wires even when devices are switched off.

The sources of electric fields we encounter and utilise daily include household or commercial wiring circuits, as well as all the devices and equipment they power. Additionally, utility cables, power lines supplying our households, power stations and substations, and distribution lines emit significant electric fields.

2. Magnetic Fields

Magnetic fields are produced by current flow. Exposure found in homes can vary considerably from one household to another. They most importantly arise from:

- Imbalances in the electric current flowing through active/hot and neutral wiring due to wiring errors or stray currents (see Chapter 9),
- The separation of active/hot and neutral cables,
- Solar panel systems and inverters,
- Electrical floor heating and
- Outside sources like power lines and transformers.

Magnetic fields penetrate most materials as if they weren't present, making shielding ineffective. The use of materials that can shield magnetic fields is costly and, in our experience, typically disappointing in a residential setting. If the source of the magnetic field cannot be mitigated, we need to increase our distance from the source.

Sources that generate magnetic fields include utility supplies, power lines, train/tram lines, and any equipment that utilises electricity for heating, cooling, or motor operation. For more information on magnetic fields, please see Chapter 2.

3. Radio Frequency

Also referred to as RF, this exists within the non-ionising band of frequencies, encompassing both radio and microwave radiation levels. Radio waves serve as carriers of information from one location to another through the air. Wireless communication infrastructures can include cell phones, phone towers, Wi-Fi routers, Bluetooth devices, radio and television broadcasts, radars, and satellites. RF can travel great distances and penetrate homes. For more information on RF, please see Chapter 3.

4. Dirty Electricity

Dirty electricity is energy that travels along household wires in buildings. This form of electronic pollution is generated by numerous modern electronic gadgets, appliances, lighting, solar systems and power solutions, LEDs, power line communication devices (PLCs), solar panel inverters, domestic appliances, switch-mode power supplies, and dimmer switches.

It's essential to note that while the source of dirty electricity may originate within your property, it can also originate from sources beyond the boundaries of your home or workplace.

Before the home assessment

Before visiting a client, I always check the proximity of nearby electrical distribution lines and cell towers relative to the house I'm scheduled to survey. I assess whether distribution lines run above the street and whether they're alongside the home or on the opposite side. I conduct a similar assessment for mobile phone towers to determine their distance from the property.

All of this provides invaluable insight into the levels of external electronic pollution in the area where the home assessment will take place.

It is essential to understand that when dealing with radio waves, it's impossible to predict the exact levels present in a location, as neighbouring buildings and their construction materials may deflect, block, or reflect radio signals towards or away from the property being assessed for EMF. Even if there are only a lot of towers in the area, their radiation could still be obstructed and attenuated by neighbouring buildings.

While conducting research beforehand can be beneficial, it's common for an actual EMF assessment inside the property to yield different results than initially anticipated. Therefore, obtaining accurate readings through an on-site assessment is crucial for understanding the level of exposure the body experiences. So, regardless of the number of cell towers in the vicinity, it's imperative to assess the interior of every room in the house, as meter readings will likely vary from room to room.

Over the years, I've found that arriving early for my survey allows me to take a brief drive around the property and explore the neighbourhood. Often, I observe details that clients may have overlooked during their years spent in the area—such as the presence of a cell tower on the rooftop of a building located only 300 metres away!

Upon arriving

Before starting, it's essential for you and the consultant to have a discussion and reach a mutual agreement on the survey's process and the objectives to be achieved upon completion. Often, these aspects may not have been discussed during the initial telephone call. It is also beneficial to reiterate the reasons for conducting the survey and to identify any specific issues or concerns.

The consultant should then provide a brief overview of the various types of radiation to be investigated in the home before outlining the survey methodology.

To ensure thoroughness during the survey, I start by reviewing the list of electrical and electronic devices and gadgets – both wired and wireless – inside the property. Below is the checklist I utilise for my surveys:

1. DECT Phone (Cordless Phone)	11. Wireless Printer	21. Smart Thermostat (Nest)
2. Microwave Oven	12. Smart Meter	22. Heating Blankets
3. Induction Cooker	13. Smart TV	23. Spring Mattress
4. IPads	14. Digital Radio Alarm clock	24. Bedside Lamps
5. Smartphones	15. Infotainment Box	25. Play / Gaming Station
6. Computers - Desk or Laptop	16. Alexa	26. WiFi Router
7. Wireless Speakers	17. Amazon Firestick	27. WiFi Booster
8. Wireless Keyboard	18. Power Line Adaptors (PLC)	28. Other
9. Wireless Mouse	19. Baby Monitors	29. Other
10. Wearable Devices	20. Wireless Camera	30. Other

After reviewing the list of electrical and electronic devices and gadgets and noting the quantity of each device (some clients, for instance, may have three to four boosters inside the house), we can proceed to start the survey.

The bedroom

The bedroom is meant to be a place where the body rests and rejuvenates. However, achieving restful and effective sleep can be challenging due to the irritation caused by various forms of EMF, including RF radiation from wireless devices and nearby cell towers, electric fields emanating from wiring within walls, and potentially magnetic fields from external distribution lines, household appliances or faulty household wiring.

Occasionally, I have observed elevated levels of magnetic fields in bedrooms situated above the kitchen or utility room or where a smart meter or consumer unit (fuse box) is positioned on the side wall adjacent to the head side of the bed. In such cases, rearranging the bed's position within the bedroom can resolve the issue.

Next, we focus on evaluating the impact of the electric field and radio frequency radiation on the body, which is of the utmost importance. During this assessment, you'll be asked to lie in bed, enabling us to accurately assess your body's exposure to both types of radiation. We'll record the highest reading obtained because peak or maximum exposure—rather than average exposure—is often the most problematic for the body.

In our industry, we advise that RF body voltage readings above 100 µV (microvolts) are considered high. If your radio frequency body readings exceed this threshold, one straightforward solution is to shield the bedroom. This can be accomplished using specialised shielding paint formulated for long-term effectiveness and suitability for health. Alternatively, you may choose to sleep under a high-quality shielding canopy.

Additionally, to mitigate the elevated levels of the electric fields on various bedroom walls, we examine the electricity distribution unit, also known as a fuse box. This unit supplies voltage to your lighting, electrical, and electronic gadgets.

By toggling circuits on and off as necessary, we can assess and identify which circuits contribute to the high electric field exposure in the bedroom, and we can reduce or eliminate the voltage – the source of the electric field – around the bedroom. For examples of verifiable and logical solutions to electric fields, please see Chapter 8.

During the assessment, we will simulate the impact of deactivating offending circuits on your body's exposure. In some but not all cases, we can eliminate the electric field in the room during sleep, allowing your body to rest and rejuvenate in an electric field-free environment throughout the night.

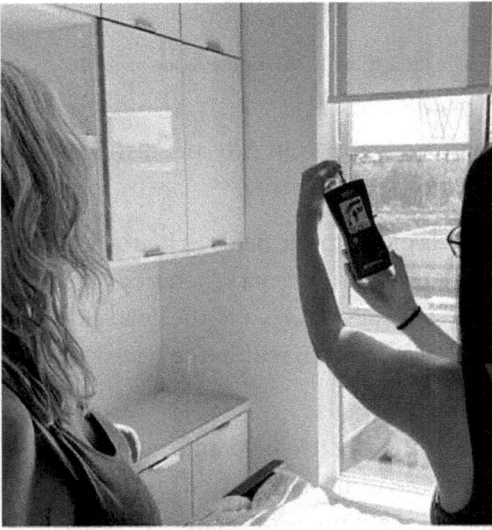

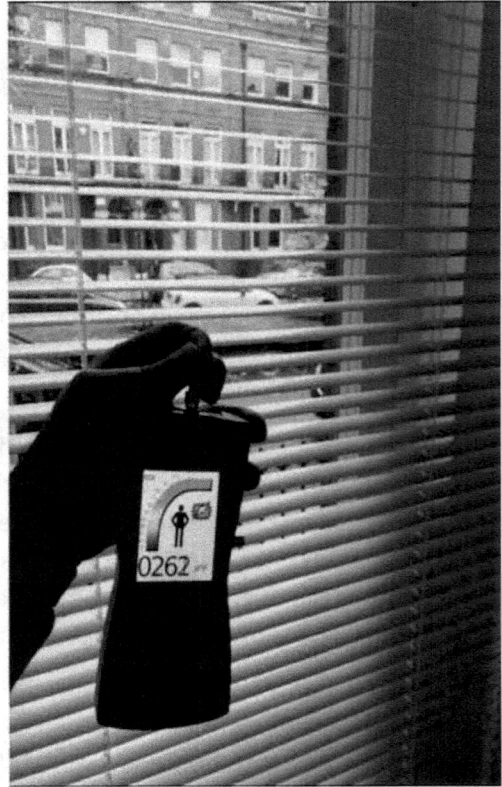

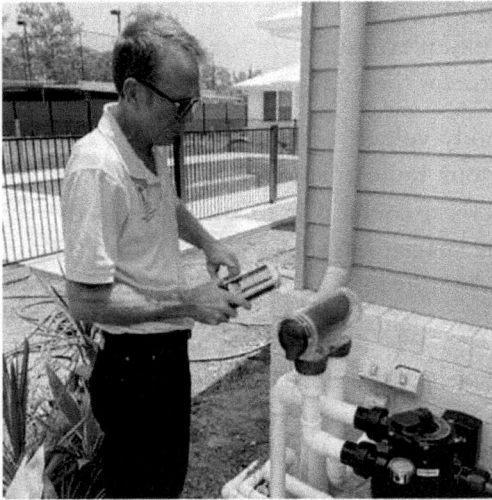

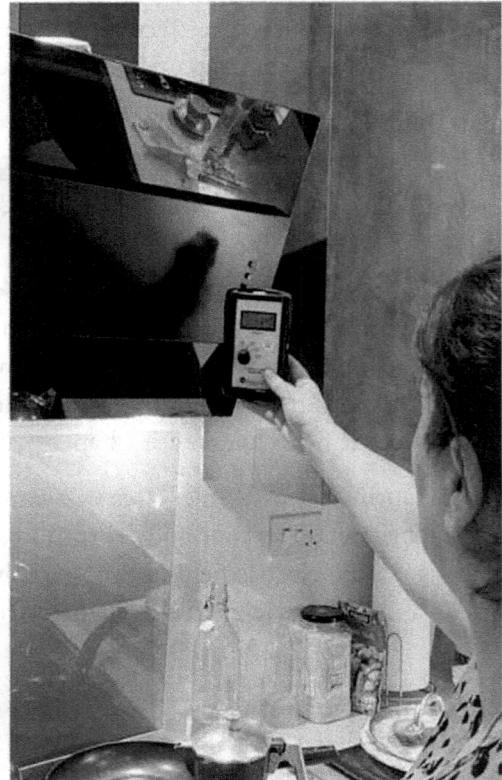

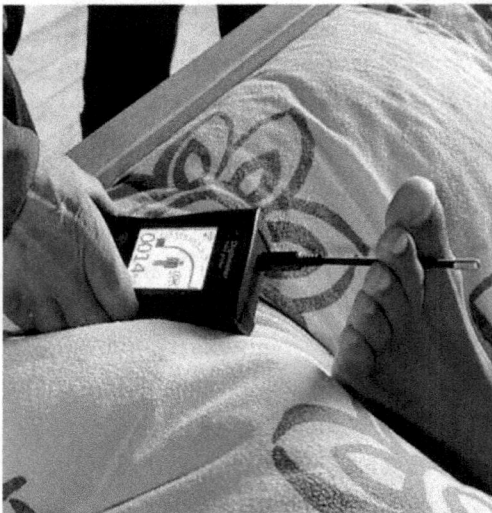

Lastly, we assess your bed. To ensure a conducive environment for rest and rejuvenation, your mattress should not produce a static magnetic field, as this can trigger stress signals in your body. Ideally, you should opt for a metal-free mattress. To determine if your mattress possesses magnetic properties, we run a compass over it. If the needle deviates by more than 5°, it is advisable to consider replacing the mattress. Additionally, choosing a metal-free mattress can help mitigate electronic pollution and other factors that may impact sleep quality. For further insights on selecting a healthy mattress, please refer to Chapter 11.

The living space

Given that you probably spend a significant portion of your day in the living room, we take its assessment seriously. If your property is situated on a main street or near or underneath an electrical distribution line, we typically encounter elevated readings just outside the property. However, as we move into the building itself, we anticipate these readings to decrease, further diminishing at the back of the property.

If high or comparable levels are detected at the back of the house, it suggests that the source of the magnetic field is likely internal, stemming from household appliances, devices, lighting (such as energy-saving spiral bulbs), or electrical faults.

Lastly, it is essential to address radio frequency radiation-emitting devices such as Wi-Fi routers, signal boosters, and infotainment boxes located near the television set. These devices should either be hardwired or shielded during the day and completely switched off at night.

The kitchen

The kitchen typically contains many electrical appliances. When these appliances are plugged into electric sockets and are in operation, electric and magnetic fields become prominent in the kitchen environment. The kitchen island, situated in the middle of some kitchens, is often powered and may also emit high levels of electric field.

We can illustrate with our instrumentation, the magnitude of the electric field absorbed by your body. Furthermore, we can demonstrate how unplugging power cables or switching off sockets can significantly reduce the electric field body reading.

Your microwave oven provides an intriguing opportunity to demonstrate how the high-frequency radiation it emits can impact you and your family. Together, we can heat something in the microwave and measure your body's absorption of RF radiation at various distances while it's in operation. This experiment will prompt you to take your safety – and that of your children, if you have any – more seriously before deciding to use your microwave in the future.

The study

These days, more and more people are working from home on laptops, tablets, or smartphones.

Here, we typically apply the same EMF assessment approach used in bedrooms and living spaces to investigate magnetic fields, and your body's absorption of electric fields and radio frequency. Based on our findings, we recommend verifiable solutions to reduce or eliminate your body's exposure to these fields.

We advocate for transitioning away from wireless technology and opting for hardwired devices wherever possible; most devices can function effectively with cables.

Summary

The journey towards a healthier home doesn't end here; this is the empowering beginning. Recognising the potential hazards of EMF in our daily lives is a crucial step, but taking action is paramount. Hiring an EMF specialist offers a bespoke solution tailored to your home's unique challenges. With their sophisticated tools and deep understanding of EMF radiation, you and the consultant can unveil nuances that lie beyond the reach of amateur assessments. Ensuring that the mitigation strategies are not just applied but optimised for your specific environment, thus safeguarding your health and enhancing the quality of your living space.

Investigating EMF presents an opportunity for empowerment and well-being. By choosing to engage a professional EMF specialist, you're not merely reacting to a potential risk; you're proactively creating a sanctuary that supports your health and peace of mind – and that of your family – based on logic and experience. And, surely, nothing is more important than your family being happy, healthy, and content in the space they call home.

When you follow the QR code, you will find additional tools to download and a way to contact me. Good luck on your journey. If I can help you, that would be wonderful.

CONNECT WITH ME

Samir Derrar
EMF Radiation Specialist, Coach

https://www.emf-hunters.com

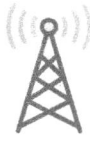

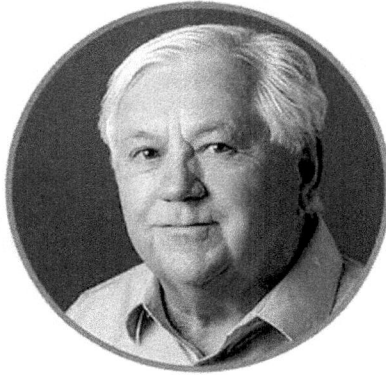

Jason R King

EMF Radiation Specialist

ABOUT THE AUTHOR: JASON R KING

Jason R. King's journey into EMF awareness and mitigation commenced when he encountered mysterious health issues potentially linked to his IT profession, working in Tampa, Florida. Constant exposure to computer monitors, electric fields from office equipment, and always-on WiFi in his work environment prompted a deep dive into researching the potentially harmful effects of EMFs on human health, particularly with the emergence of 5G technology.

As the 5G infrastructure was being rolled out by the telecoms industry in the Tampa Bay area of Florida and nationwide, Jason began engaging actively with advocacy groups such as Americans for Safe Technology and The US Brain Tumor Association, co-founding and producing the informative platform 5Ginformation.net. This initiative aimed to raise awareness about EMFs and address public safety concerns. Additionally, he played a pivotal role in organizing concerned citizens in Florida, uniting electrically sensitive individuals, Florida residents, and EMF practitioners for collaborative efforts.

Driven by a quest for solutions, Jason pursued training at the renowned GEOVITAL Academy in Melbourne, Australia, and the GEOVITAL Akademie für Naturheilkunde und Strahlenschutz in Austria. These institutions, with over 40 years of experience in environmental health, equipped him with expertise to establish an EMF mitigation practice.

Transitioning from his personal wellness challenges to public advocacy, Jason founded his consultancy at emfgeo.com. Through this platform, he provides guidance and practical solutions to individuals interested in understanding EMF exposure, who are concerned about its impacts, or suffering from Electromagnetic Hypersensitivity (EHS).

Prior to his EMF consultancy, Jason had a rich background spanning over three decades in the IT sector, focusing on Design, Marketing, and Visual Communications, where he contracted with companies like IBM, Lotus Software, Verizon, and others, across many diverse markets.

Now as the owner of EMFGEO dba / KingGroup Solutions LLC, Jason serves as an EMF consultant in the Tampa Bay area of Florida, USA. For those seeking assistance in navigating EMF concerns or exploring protective measures for their living spaces, Jason can be reached through the QR code provided.

Jason's dedication to promoting EMF awareness and providing practical solutions underscores his commitment to enhancing public health and safety in an increasingly digital world.

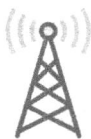

CHAPTER 6

LITTLE THINGS YOU CAN DO YOURSELF TO REDUCE EMF AT HOME

By Jason R King

I'm glad you're here and are taking steps to safeguard yourself and your family from EMF radiation exposure. In this Chapter, I'll share several strategies you can implement immediately to reduce EMF radiation in your home and from your phone.

It's important to understand that while these tips can help lower your exposure, they alone cannot create a completely healthy environment. To achieve a truly restful and restorative space, you'll need the assistance of an experienced, qualified professional. This expert can use specialized meters to assess your home's EMF impact on your body, not just the air, and then work with you to implement comprehensive mitigation measures.

As you read through these initial tips, remember that they are a good starting point, but further action will be required to address EMF exposure in your living space fully—especially the sleeping area, which is the most important room for your health.

This section provides helpful tips and practical, simple steps for the most common situations. You can understand their application more deeply from many of the other chapters in this book and by contacting any of our colleagues published here.

Let's dive into the steps you can take right now to reduce your EMF levels.

Why are we concerned about EMF Radiation?

Emf's exist within a range of frequencies, with higher frequencies having shorter wavelengths and lower frequencies having longer wavelengths. Some of the familiar EMF sources we are concerned with are classified as non-ionizing radiation, with most of our exposure being from man-made electronics. Although non-ionizing radiation (radiation with a lower frequency than visible light) is considered safe by government bodies and the tech/telecoms industries, IARC, a body of the WHO, does classify low-frequency EMFs as a "possible human carcinogen." Emerging research has found that our cells' proteins (VGCCs) are disrupted, leading to oxidative stress, DNA damage, and apoptosis (cell death). As well the INTERPHONE study points to brain cancer linked to the high use of cell phones.

Most of us are precautionary here; if you want to familiarize yourself with more scientific research that critiques our established assumptions, start with the BioInitiative Report and the work of Dr. Martin L Pall, Martin Blank, Ph.D., Dr. Olle Johansson, and Dr.Magda Havas, Ph.D. But for now, let's move on to our main objective for practical and preventative solutions.

Understanding Electromagnetic Hypersensitivity (EHS)

Electromagnetic hypersensitivity (EHS) is becoming a modern-day health concern experienced by many people. This is driving increased awareness about the potential health impacts of electromagnetic radiation (EMR). As a result, many individuals are now seeking ways to reduce their exposure to EMR and lead a healthier life.

Symptoms of Electromagnetic Hypersensitivity

EHS is a recognized medical diagnosis that is becoming more prevalent each year. Some of the commonly reported symptoms associated with exposure to radio frequency (RF) radiation are:

- Fatigue, stress, agitation, anxiety, irritability

- Insomnia, sleep problems

- Headaches/migraines, memory or learning problems

- Depression/anxiety

- Tinnitus (ringing in ears)

- Visual disruption/light sensitivity

- Heart palpitations/dizziness

We all want to avoid these unwanted health impacts, so let's go through a few easy precautions and a good starting point for cleaning up EMFs in your home.

As a general rule in the home, take these steps:

- Eliminate, Reduce, and Distance yourself from any source that's emitting EMFs.

- Don't use Microwave ovens, or leave the room when you do! Surprisingly, Microwaves that heat food can travel well over 40 feet or more into your living areas when they are in operation.

- Replace your Microwave oven with safer conventional appliances such as a toaster oven or a traditional range.

- To lessen electric fields from energized electrical appliances, add timers or manual switches to turn off lights, TVs, or entertainment centers at your power outlets and switch them off when unnecessary.

- Check all power outlets in your home for proper grounding with a ground tester. Outlet testers have color-coded guides to confirm if they are properly grounded. If the tester shows they are not grounded correctly, get a licensed electrician to fix them.

- Avoid dimmer switches or any dimmable device, as they may produce transient voltage and can create magnetic fields. Regular on-off switches are preferred, as they do not have this problem. Laptop chargers, solar inverters, and smart meters have similar issues.

- Replace DECT / digital cordless phones (they emit high RF radiation at all times) with corded landlines.

- Unplug electric appliances, such as radios/alarm clocks, stereos, heating pads, and electric blankets, to cease electric and magnetic field emissions.

- Avoid using compact fluorescent lights (CFLs) and other low-voltage lighting technologies. They emit high levels of potentially harmful electromagnetic radiation. For safer lighting options, use incandescent bulbs or 120-volt halogen bulbs instead.

Protecting Children from EMF Exposure

Children, in particular, are more vulnerable due to their young bodies' smaller size and bone density. For instance, the Agency for Research on Cancer states that children can absorb up to 10 times more wireless radiation in the bone marrow of their skull compared to adults. Studies also link childhood Leukemia to nearby radio stations, high-voltage power lines, and high-EMF environments.

Limit your child's internet use to Ethernet-wired devices; you can achieve this with "dongles" that adapt to Ethernet connections. Any device should have its WiFi and Bluetooth settings disabled until you need the connection. Ensure your kids use a laptop or computer on a table, not on their laps or resting on any part of their bodies.

Please set up a dedicated Children's desk with Ethernet connectivity where they can be observed. Keep those power cords (use three-pronged) away from their feet, just as you should do in your own home office. Use an external wired keyboard/mouse when possible.

Set limits for their screen time to a specific time of day and not for at least 1 1/2 hours before bedtime. Place more importance on other activities that are not digitally available, such as board games, building model cars, sports, and other outdoor activities with you, the parent, such as nature walks and gardening.

Choose a Low-EMF Baby Monitor

Suppose you have a child and use a baby monitor. In that case, there are some essential steps you can take to minimize their exposure to EMF radiation.

Instead of a wireless connection, connect the baby monitor to your home network using an Ethernet cable. This wired setup will significantly reduce the EMF emissions compared to a wireless system. If you are unwilling to move away from being connected via WiFi, place the baby monitor as far away from your child's crib or bed as possible. Maximizing the distance between the device and your child's sleeping area can help minimize their exposure. Even placing an aluminum foil barrier between the bedroom unit and the child can reduce its impact.

It's important to note that babies and children are even more vulnerable to the potential health effects of EMFs than adults. The WHO also puts radiofrequency radiation in the same category as exhaust fumes. Please take these precautions to protect your little one from unnecessary EMF exposure.

Tips Summary:

- Avoid all "Smart" toys that incorporate WiFi or Bluetooth.

- Always choose wired options when possible.

- Please only give your child a smartphone at an appropriate age, then set rules for their use.

- Limit screen time and use wired Ethernet connections with Ethernet adapters and dongles on your tablets and computers.

- Seek helpful organizations like the Baby Safe Project and Healthy Tech Home for guidance on tech and kids.

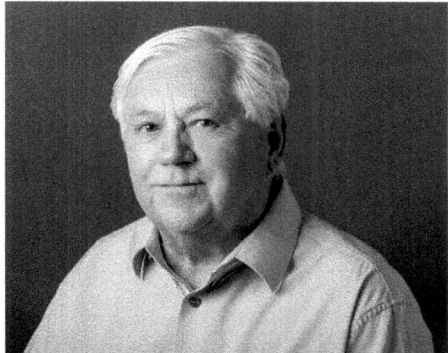

Photo of Jason R King

Routers and Home Networks

When minimizing your exposure to electromagnetic radiation (EMR) from wireless devices, your WiFi router is an important consideration. Here are some tips to help you reduce your EMR exposure from your home WiFi setup:

Position Your Router Strategically

Please ensure your WiFi router is as far from your living, working, and sleeping spaces as possible. The strength of RF radiation decreases with distance, so the further you can be from the router, the better; place WiFi-enabled routers as far away as possible from the areas where you and your family spend the most time.

Switch to a Wired Home Network

Switching from wireless to wired connections is one of the most effective ways to reduce RF radiation exposure in your home. Here's how you can create a high-speed, wired home network:

Use Wired Ethernet Connections

Replace wireless connections with wired Ethernet wherever possible. Gigabit Ethernet switches and shielded CAT-7 cables can help you build a robust wired network infrastructure in your home.

Invest in Wired Network Equipment

When it's time to upgrade your internet equipment, consider purchasing a compatible modem or wired non-WiFi router rather than relying on the all-in-one devices provided by your cable company. A "wired-first" approach will give you more control over your home network.

Turn Off the WiFi When Sleeping

If you use WiFi, consider turning off your router while sleeping for an even better night's sleep. You can accomplish this in several ways:

- Physically unplug the router before bed and plug it back in when you wake up. This is a free and straightforward solution.

- **Remote-Controlled Switch:** To turn the router off and on, use an infrared outlet switch (not a WiFi or Bluetooth-controlled switch).

- **Outlet Timer:** Install an outlet timer that switches the WiFi router off at bedtime and back on in the morning.

Implementing one of these shutdown methods and strategically positioning your WiFi router can significantly reduce your EMR exposure from WiFi.

To recap, here are some of the top tips;

- Do not use WiFi; use Ethernet cable only. Network your home; it will be worth it in the end.

- If WiFi is enabled, turn off your internet routers at night when not in use (use a timer or power switch)

- If using WiFi, reduce the power density with your router settings or cover the router with RF shielding fabric.

- Use shielded and grounded cabling when possible and three-prong plugs on all your computers and devices.

- Use external wired keyboards and mice on your computers.

Being "Smart" about your Smart Home

When selecting new smart home devices, security systems, appliances, and other electronics, vital considerations include reducing RF radiation exposure in your living space. Prioritizing wired connections and strategic placement can create a healthier environment with reduced EMF exposure.

Opt for Non-Wireless Models

Choose appliances and devices that do not have built-in WiFi or Bluetooth connectivity. Choose devices that support wired Ethernet connections (use shielded Ethernet cables to connect these devices) instead of wireless. If those wireless features are present, inquire about the ability to disable them if you don't plan on using them.

Entertainment systems

To avoid the EMF emissions from their wireless radios, use wired speakers only or speakers connected via Ethernet instead of Bluetooth or WiFi.

Strategic Placement of Wireless Devices

If you have wireless devices like a WiFi router, place them as far away as possible from the areas where you and your family spend the most time. This helps minimize your exposure to the high EMF levels these devices can produce.

Implement Automatic Shutoffs

Consider using timers or switches to automatically turn off wireless devices like traditional WiFi routers and smart speakers when they are not in use, especially overnight.

Mobile Phones and Radiation Harms

Keep this in mind when using your mobile phone; it's from Apple's own iPhone manual:

"When using an iPhone near your body for voice calls or wireless data transmission over a cellular network, keep the iPhone at least 15 mm (5/8 inch) away from the body, and only use carrying cases, belt clips, or holders that do not have metal parts and that maintain at least 15 mm (5/8 inch) separation between the iPhone and the body."

They probably didn't tell you that when you purchased your phone at an Apple Store.

Next, I would like you to learn how your phone is tested for what they call "safety" on a plastic dummy that is a 6ft 2in 220lb male model. Unfortunately, there is no SAM "Phantom" for pregnant women or children.

You can learn more about SAM at this advocacy website, *We Are Not Sam*, at https://www.wearenotsam.com/

You may recall if you're of a certain age that back in the day when smoking in public was an acceptable practice, the Tobacco industry claimed there was no linkage to cancer from smoking. Over time and with millions of dollars spent in lawsuits, the linkage to cancer has been established, and not only from smoking tobacco itself but secondhand exposure as well.

Now, please consider that radiofrequency radiation from Telecom facilities, mobile phones, and WiFi is the new secondhand smoke.

Every phone model has a SAR (specific absorption rate) ranking, which results from testing using the "SAM Phantom." The higher the SAR rating, the more radiation is absorbed into your body. Knowing this, you may choose a phone with the lowest possible SAR rating. However, the best option is not to use or limit the use of your cell phone and maintain a safe distance from the device when in use.

Remember that The FCC guidelines for SAR testing allow for a separation distance (remember the iPhone manual warning?) between the phone and the user that may not reflect how most people use their devices.

The Environmental Working Group (EWG) puts it into perspective here:

"The FCC's cell phone radiation standards closely follow the 1992 recommendations of the Institute of Electrical and Electronics Engineers (IEEE) (FCC 1997). These standards allow 20 times more radiation to penetrate the head than the rest of the body and do not account for risks to children."

So, let's be honest about industry and government standards: Sadly, they are outdated and do not accurately reflect real-world conditions.

Reducing EMF Exposure from Your Smartphone

Knowing that your smartphone can be a significant EMF radiation source, here are several steps you can take to minimize your exposure:

- Use Airplane Mode and disable Bluetooth and Wifi

- When you're not actively using your phone for calls or data, enable the "Airplane Mode" feature. This will shut off the cellular, WiFi, and Bluetooth radios, significantly reducing your device's EMF emissions.

- Check your phone settings to ensure Bluetooth and WiFi are genuinely off. Consider changing your default Bluetooth and WiFi settings to "off" and only enable it when needed. The quick-access Bluetooth control on iPhones doesn't entirely turn off the Bluetooth radio, so you'll need to go into your phone's settings to toggle it off completely.

- Remember to check your settings after software updates, as they may turn Bluetooth back on.

Optimize Call Habits

Keep the device as far from your head when making phone calls.

- Use the speakerphone or a set of "air tube" headphones to create distance between the phone and your body.

- Avoid making calls when you have a weak signal, as your phone will need to work harder to maintain the connection, increasing EMF output.

These simple adjustments can significantly reduce your overall EMF exposure and create a less harmful relationship with your mobile technology. But keep in mind: It's not a panacea.

Additional Tips

In light of what you have just learned, consider these preventative measures as well:

- Always keep your phone off your body; no direct contact with the skin.

- Don't store your phone in your pockets. Even in flight mode, it remains an electrical device.

- Only power on your phone when needed. Your phone emits radiation as long as it's on, so reduce use and increase distance.

- Use a headset ('Air Tube' recommended); never place the phone against your head.

- Don't use Airpods; Airpods and wireless earbuds also emit wireless radiofrequency radiation.

- Keep your phone off the body in an RF reduction phone case or pouch. Exposure to RF-EMR has been linked to lower sperm count in men and could compromise women's ability to conceive.

- Use airplane mode when not using your phone, then enable it when you want to collect messages or place a call.

- Keep your phone off the nightstand where you sleep and away from you when charging.

- Use a phone VIOP service from your internet provider or services like Google Voice to forward calls to your computer when you're home, so you don't have to use your mobile.

- DECT or cordless phones, like cell phones, have radiation risks, too. Use an actual landline or try a VOIP phone service instead from your internet provider. Services like Google Voice can also forward calls to your computer when you're home, so you don't have to use your mobile.

Sleeping areas

Sleeping areas are critical for your health. For eight hours a day, for your entire life, you are in a room that should be all about rest and restoration; keeping that environment as protected as possible with low to no EMFs should be your number one goal.

- Be mindful of charging stations. Do not place clocks or radios on the nightstand, as they give off surprisingly strong EMF as long as they are plugged in. Move them further away or convert them to battery power.

- In our experience, the electric fields on the bedroom wall are likely too high (your EMF consultant can help you determine if that's the case). It would be best to deal with this exposure by properly investigating which circuits are responsible and terminating those during sleep time.

- You can turn off the room's circuit at the fuse box with an adequately installed circuit cut-off switch (electrician installation required). Switching circuit breakers off manually is a safety concern and is not recommended.

- Consider RF shielding paint for the entire bedroom or an RF or shielding canopy for the bed. For more information, refer to Chapters 7 and 8.

Home office

Home offices usually contain power cords, computers, printers, and phones. It's tough to get it all under control, so tackle one thing at a time.

- Arrange power station charger locations for your phones and devices away from the body.

- Use RF shielding pads for laptops and RF shielding pouches for cell phones.

- Remove, disable, or turn off devices (printers, scanners, fax machines) that use Bluetooth signals when not needed (that's also RF).

- Keep all office equipment and computers powered by grounded three-pronged cables.

- Ethernet everything instead of WiFi.

Traveling

When traveling, we are often surrounded by many RF signals and Wi-Fi networks, which can be overwhelming. To make things easier, try implementing some of these tips to lighten the load:

- Hotels–Unplug those nightstand alarm clocks and bring a piece of shielding fabric to make a temporary canopy over the bed for sleeping in your room.

- Cars–Of course, never use your mobile while driving, but check your car's instrumentation settings to turn off Bluetooth; chances are it's always on.

- Limit Cell Phone use in cars–the car's metal surfaces intensify the RF radiation through multiple reflections.

- Navigation–If you're using maps on your mobile, you can gather the data for your trip in the map app and then put your phone in airplane mode, and it will work just fine.

Evaluating a new property or living place

Before putting money down on an apartment or home, ensure your EMF requirements are met!

- When buying property or renting a new home, be aware of where smart meters and circuit breaker panels are placed (not against your bedroom), where power lines or transformers are located (not on your side of the street), and have no mobile towers within your line of sight, and as far away as possible.

- See: https://www.antennasearch.com/ or https://www.cellmapper.net/

- The most indispensable recommendation when buying property or renting a new living place is to ensure your magnetic field readings are well below 1mG, with 0.3 or less preferred for sleeping at night. You can detect this with a TriField TF2 meter. See Chapter 4.

- If you're buying a property, buy a TriField TF2 meter and go to the property to get readings at different times of the day and night (!) before you decide. Once you have decided the magnetic field readings are acceptable, contact one of our qualified consultants for a more extensive property evaluation.

Now that you have some basic strategies to lighten the EMF burden, use the free checklist (link below) to take a survey of your home. Again, these tips alone do not completely get you out of harm's way. Remember that the biggest priority for EMF radiation for you and your family is to get the sleeping environment right, which you will need assistance with; if I can assist you with that, let me know.

To help you on your way, follow the QR code for links to many of the sources mentioned in this chapter and download a free EMF checklist.

Jason R King
EMFGEO.COM

CONNECT WITH ME

Jason R King
EMF Radiation Specialist

https://emfgeo.com/emfbooktips

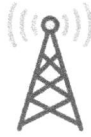

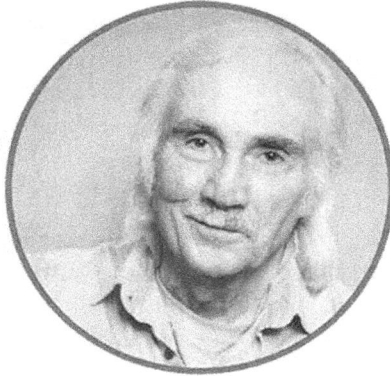

Marcus Schluschen

EMF Radiation Specialist, Geobiologist,
Activist, Photographer

ABOUT THE AUTHOR:
MARCUS SCHLUSCHEN

Marcus Schluschen is an experienced EMF radiation consultant in the Vancouver and Vancouver Island region of British Columbia, Canada. Before he became a certified EMF consultant, he would have never considered that one day he would be communicating with scientists and physicians from around the world and helping translate peer-reviewed medical research papers on radiation exposure from his native German to English.

Marcus's expertise in EMF home assessment and radiation mitigation led to several public speaking engagements. His greatest reward is when clients who have had little success with other approaches to health call to report that they are finally sleeping well again and that their health is steadily improving.

Through the health struggles of a close family member, Marcus witnessed how chronic, non-ionizing radiation exposure carries inherent risks, leading to needless suffering and declining health.

He experienced how life can rapidly turn upside down when a loved one became afflicted by electro-hypersensitivity (EHS), which had devastating impacts on their life.

Marcus enrolled in a professional radiation consulting course with the GEOVITAL Academy for Radiation Protection and Geobiology in Austria to learn how to protect his family and advise others on how to protect themselves.

He attended the 4-day International EMF Medical Conference 2021, where he learned about needless human suffering from involuntary, chronic EMF radiation exposure in today's technology-saturated world, affecting young and old.

Marcus volunteers in a long-term global science project on the increase of non-ionizing radiation exposure emanating from modern technologies in communities and the environment. He supports anti-cell tower movements in communities and successfully helped public opposition against cell towers in residential neighbourhoods.

Being a lover of the art of photography, Marcus studied professional photography and has spent over 30 years creating photo images for magazines, publications, businesses, and private individuals. He enjoys reading good books and loves being in nature with his classic film camera, creating black-and-white fine art photographs, which he develops in his traditional darkroom.

For a home assessment, please get in touch with Marcus at www.radiationfreelife.com .

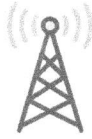

CHAPTER 7

EMF MITIGATION - SHIELDING PAINT

By Marcus Schluschen

Welcome to this chapter on shielding paint, about protection and the goal of maintaining good health.

Unlike our forefathers, we live in a time of unprecedented involuntary radiation exposure from an ever-growing array of wireless technologies, all while governments lay claim to protecting the public. Incredibly, none of their safety claims seem to stand up to independent scientific scrutiny, as they are based on thermal heating of the body only.

Over the years, public radiation exposure has been steadily on the rise, while today's exposure levels of citizens inside their homes have risen dramatically, without anyone's informed consent.

In this chapter, we focus on the use of shielding paint and its dual function to mitigate radiofrequency radiation (RF), and electric field pollution (EF), which is found in excessive levels in nearly every home.

Protect yourself and your loved ones.

Protecting homes with shielding paint has been proven successful worldwide and used by many families, as well as informed architects and designers of high-end homes, luxury condos, and prestigious hotels.

If you are planning a renovation of your current home or feel the need to protect yourself and your family from today's relentless electrosmog exposure, this chapter will provide you with fundamental knowledge to create a safer home.

Investigate, Avoid, Eliminate and Shield

The first step to a safer home is to identify, avoid, and eliminate all possible sources of electronic pollution inside your home. Please refer to Chapters 2 and 3 for radiation sources and learn how to investigate this in Chapters 4 and 5.

NOTE: We do not advise anyone to start a shielding project without a proper home assessment by a well-trained EMF consultant with superior instrumentation and understanding of how to holistically mitigate unwelcome electronic pollution in your home. If painting walls and ceilings are not an option, other creative possibilities exist.

When working with a consultant, you will learn where the problematic areas in your house are and receive guidance and solutions to effectively and safely mitigate electrosmog pollution in your home. Please refer to Chapter 5.

Using the right shielding paint to protect your home is not exclusively the only requirement to turn a bedroom into a sleep sanctuary, as other factors might need to be weighted, which could potentially make you decide not to shield and consider moving.

There are several ways of protecting against EMFs, which can be achieved through;

- Shielding paint - applied to walls, ceilings, window and door frames, cabinets, etc.

- Shielding mesh - often used on floors, behind drywall, and under roof tiles.

- RF protective fabric - used for window covering, door openings, partitions, and as bed canopies.

Adding value to your home

Shielding adds value to your home if you consider selling it in the future.

More and more people appreciate a low EMF environment, and holistically designed solutions can be attractive for health-orientated buyers.

Bedrooms – the most important rooms to protect in your home.

Choosing Shielding Paint

There are several shielding paints on the market, including cheap varieties. As with any project, low-cost options are rarely conducive to achieving optimal results. Choosing high-quality products to create a healthier environment provides peace of mind and presents the best you can do for your family.

GEOVITAL's T98 shielding paint achieved exceptional RF reduction results in countless homes, and due to its outstanding holistic compatibility with people, it is always highly recommended by informed health practitioners when not only shielding but also long-term health compatibility in general is of importance.

Considering we are trying to create the best solutions for a healthy environment that agrees with the resident's long-term health on many levels, I feel it also maximizes the holistic goal we want to achieve.

Most people want a good solution to their situation, not an experiment.

The development of protective measures against radiofrequency radiation began in 1998 with the arrival of commercial wireless communication for the general population. T98 shielding paint was developed with a focus on self-application by patients with varying health problems. This means this is not industrial paint, as is often offered on the Internet, but shielding paint specially developed with wellness in mind to include patients with intolerances. Allergic reactions or other problems should not occur in this user group, which is often the case with industrial shielding paints!

It is a highly effective shielding paint against radio frequency radiation from sources such as mobile phone towers, directional radio, radar, airport

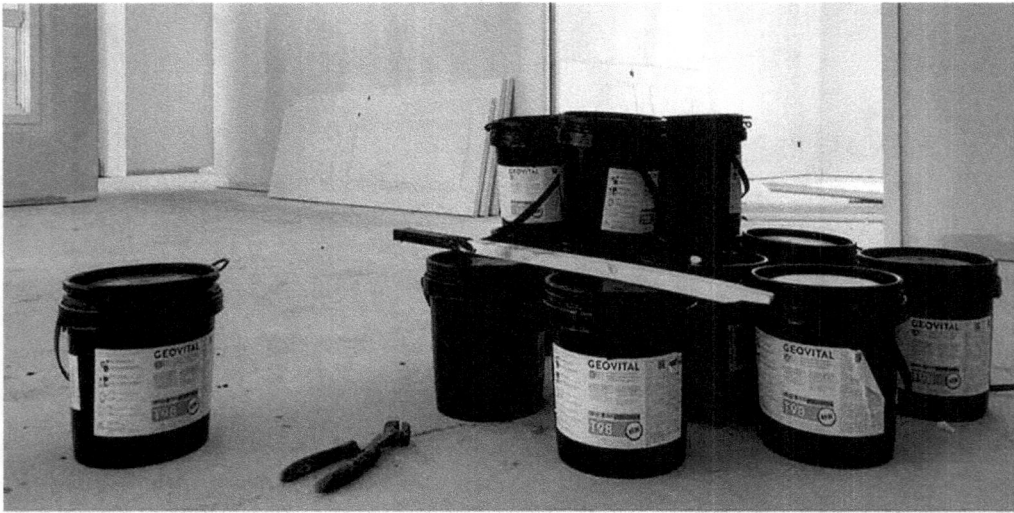

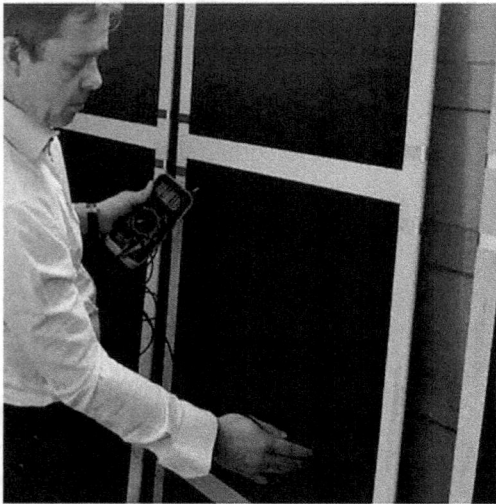

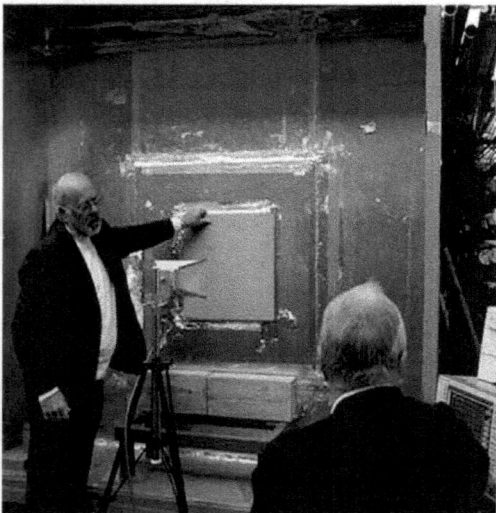

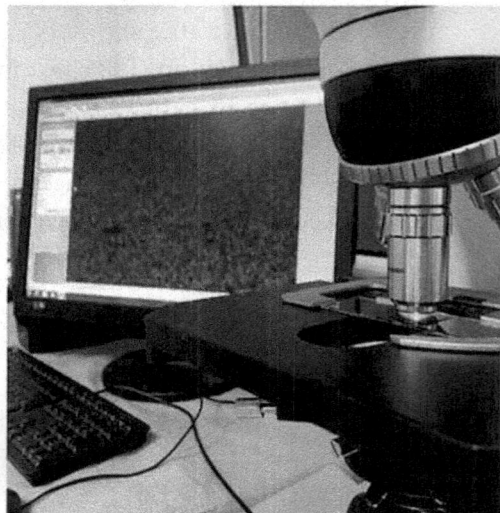

This protective paint was regularly tested, independently at the Bundeswehr (military) University lab in Munich, Germany, by Professor Pauli. While

GEOVITAL, of course, conducts its own internal testing for quality control and to develop regular improvements to the product, it never relied on in-house testing alone.

The outstanding feature of this paint is that it is carbon-based, breathable, solvent-free, with extremely low Volatile Organic Compounds (VOC) emissions, but it is GEOVITAL's aim to avoid allergic and intolerance reactions, which makes it ideal for holistic home protection.

Shielding Paint Functions

Shielding paint turns walls, ceilings, and other surfaces into barriers that keep radiofrequency radiation and electric fields at bay. The shielding properties, however, do not extend to magnetic fields, from sources like transmission, or street power lines. A positive feature of T98 is that natural Earth signals seem to pass through unobstructed.

Shielding paint partially absorbs but predominantly deflects RF radiation. A very small amount comes through. It is important to know that both sides of the paint deflect RF radiation, similar to how a double-sided mirror reflects light on both sides.

This paint also blocks low-frequency electric fields from electrical wiring, when grounded. Electric fields are attracted to ground, so when the paint sits between you and the electric field source and is properly grounded, the electric fields will leave via the paint and not enter your living space.

Shielding paint can be used inside the home as well as outside, but it must be covered.

If used outside, it cannot protect well against electric fields on the inside. When this paint is used outside, your EMF consultant can brief you on its application and grounding options.

Is it difficult to apply shielding paint?

Anyone should be able to shield their bedroom with shielding paint, and it is so easy that it can be accomplished over a weekend.

- It handles like regular paint, except that you use a thick, fuzzy paint roller that gives the paint a slightly different texture.

- Shielding paint does require frequent stirring to ensure the paint ingredients remain suspended before topping up your paint tray.

- Since the paint is black, a quality primer paint is required before applying a finish coat in the colour of your choice.

What should be shielded?

When deciding where to shield, remember that shielding paint predominantly deflects RF radiation, and that typically, cell tower radiation comes from different directions. You might have a tower closer to you, which is your main concern, but others are also reaching you from other sides.

The most common mistake - shielding a single bedroom wall.

Since shielding paint reflects on both sides, which causes other signals on your side of the wall to bounce back into the room, you receive them twice, once directly and a second time via deflection from the paint which can end up nearly doubling your exposure from other sources on your side of the wall. Therefore, shielding a single wall would unlikely achieve what a body RF assessment would confirm to be a desirable result.

Bedroom shielding paint basics

An easy way to create a healthier sleeping environment, where your body can rejuvenate, is to paint a room completely with shielding paint on the inside, essentially creating a Faraday cage.

- Shield all walls and the ceiling around you.

- On the ground level, you should not be affected by RF from below and may not need to shield the floor.

- However, if your home is elevated, and RF or electric fields are coming in from below, such as in apartments or condos, shielding mesh on the floor would be required.

- Paint bathroom doors and frames where needed.

- Ideally, paint the inside of the closet and the door frame; alternatively, paint the door(s) and frame.

- Use shielding fabric to cover windows.

Why not add shielding - if your home needs repainting?

How many layers of shielding paint are required?

It all depends on the quality and effectiveness of the shielding paint you choose. Cheaper paints may require extra layers to accomplish similar result. However, shielding effectiveness is not the only benchmark, as you also want a healthy home, so not all ingredients are justified in your journey for a safer home.

With T98 paint, a two-layer application was a standard recommendation for the longest time. Today, with more and stronger RF sources, this is frequently no longer enough, and three layers have become the norm. In years to come, 6G will have made its debut and four layers are expected to be needed.

Each layer brings you back about seven years, relative to your exposure. Two layers would bring you back to how your exposure was 14 years ago, and three would represent 21 years.

Instead of adding more shielding later, add the layers now, while the work is being done, as its an easy, cost-effective buffer for the future.

NOTE: When shielding against electric fields only, a single layer of shielding paint will suffice, but grounding tape still requires shielding paint on both sides.

How to prepare and apply shielding

Let your EMF consultant know when you or your painter will apply the shielding paint so that he/she can be available for questions. This guide will be helpful, but you will likely want to know more, and seeking advice from a consultant familiar with your situation will go a long way in avoiding costly mistakes.

General suggestions and tips that may be useful:

- Order floor shielding materials if needed and plan where the ground connection should be made. Run the tape from the lower part of the wall, down the baseboard, right to the floor, and leave enough tape so a firm connection to the shielding mesh and its strapping can be made.

- Move furniture out of the room or place it covered in the center if you can work around it.

- Clean walls and degrease if possible.

- Give surfaces a light sanding. Be careful in older homes, as lead paint may be present. Consult a local paint store on how to test for lead. If it's lead paint, the recommendation is not to disturb it—do not sand!

- Paint the ceiling and walls – painting edges/corners with a brush before using the roller.

- Do not paint shielding paint right up to electrical outlets, light switches, or ceiling lights, but leave a space of approximately 5 cm / 2 inches around it.

- When shielding the floor, painting the baseboards is recommended.

- If the floor does not need shielding, many prefer not to shield the baseboards.

- Shield doors, window frames and mouldings to avoid gaps in your shielding as much as possible.

- Shielded doors do not require grounding.

- Use shielding fabric over doors and windows or unshielded wood-work, but make sure to overlap the paint by about 10 cm / 4 inches.

- Ventilate well during the painting and drying process.

- Stir very well with a 'paint mixing drill' attachment before using the paint. A stir stick will work, but requires effort to mix thoroughly. Give the paint a light stir whenever you are ready to top up your paint tray, or the working ingredients will settle to the bottom of the pail, causing uneven application.

- For built-in closets, shield the inside, which can be grounded and protected against electric fields. If it is difficult due to shelving, shield the back of closet doors or consider hanging a panel of NOVA shielding fabric in front of the doors, which can be opened in the morning.

- Avoid using a paint sprayer, as it might clog up the nozzle.

- Shielding paint can be used on the floor, but mesh is preferred.

Note: Metal roofs do not negate the need to shield ceilings, due to gaps/space between the roof and walls.

Applying grounding tape

Shielding paint is highly conductive and could potentially pose a health risk if electricity accidentally comes in contact with this paint, by perhaps nailing into the wall and hitting electrical wiring. Grounding is a safety feature that allows your circuit breakers to cut the power instantly.

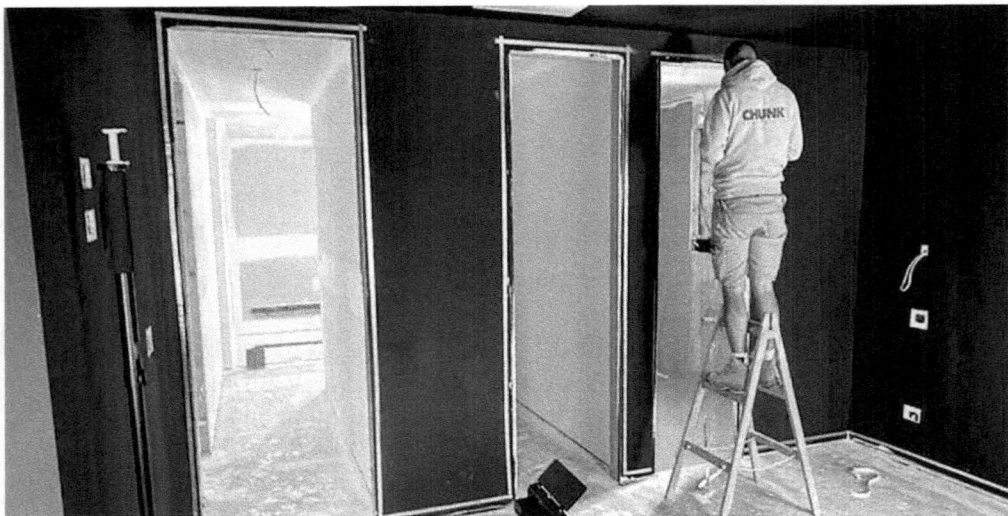

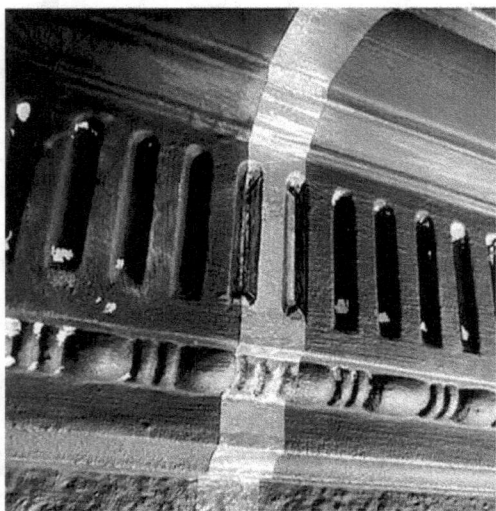

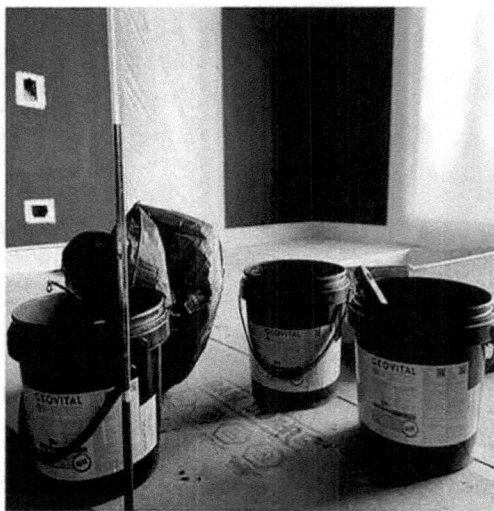

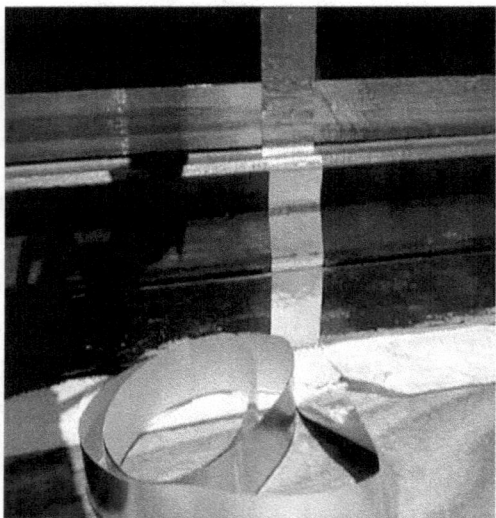

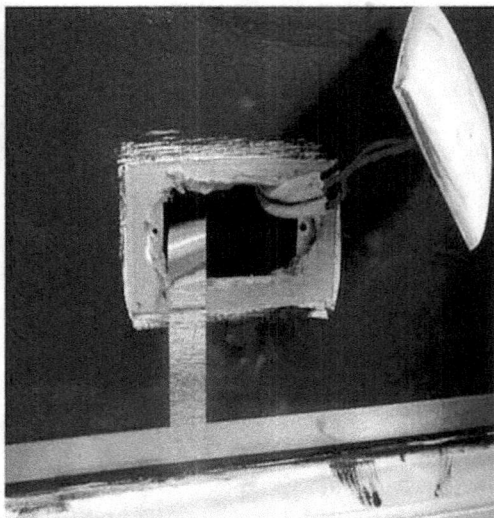

Grounding tape is typically applied just above the baseboards. L-shaped corners and T-junctions can be made by sticking the tape on top of itself and changing direction, routing towards an outlet for grounding or the floor to connect with floor shielding. When leading the tape into the cavity of an outlet, it is best to aim near the side of the outlet rather than directly at where the electrical wiring might be.

Leave the backing of the tape on and push about 30 cm / 1 foot into the outlet so the electrician has enough material to work with when completing the ground connection.

For aesthetic and safety reasons, we do not recommend using grounding plates, as they might raise questions and disappointment if the home is being sold.

Also, grounding plates with power cords that have to be plugged into the electrical outlet for ground connection is a bad idea, as grounding is an important safety feature and should never be accidentally disconnected and forgotten.

Routing the tape directly into the outlet is tidy, safer, and cheaper.

GEOVITAL's grounding tape has a brushed surface to which paint adheres. Its electrically conductive adhesive allows for ground connection from both sides.

NOTE: Do not use grounding tape 'without electrically conductive adhesive' as this will insulate, meaning proper grounding cannot be accomplished.

The tape leaves a clean finish, and since this conductive metal tape is not made of fibers, it does not increase in length and forms waves or bubbles when overpainted too generously. While thin, the grounding tape can still be noticed when covered by paint, so it's best to run it just above the baseboard.

Grounding tape comes in 10, 20, or 30-meter rolls (33, 66, or 100 feet). The 10-meter roll is good for a spare, but large rolls allow for less waste and fewer joints.

When the flow of the tape around the room is interrupted by a door, you can go around the door frame and over the top, but this might not look agreeable if the tape is located in a highly visible location. Instead, you can discontinue the tape on one side of the door and start a new tape on the other side. As the tape is now interrupted, you may have to connect to the ground in two locations, as unconnected tape serves no purpose. When connecting to the ground in two outlets, ensure they share the same electrical circuit.

The typical choice is to ground in an outlet. Alternatively, your electrician could create a dedicated ground connection for all shielded rooms. Ask your consultant for guidance.

ALWAYS use a licensed electrician to make the ground connection.

How to deal with window protection

NOVA fabric is an attractive product with great shielding performance and an excellent choice for window covering.

When shielding windows, overlap unpainted surfaces with shielding fabric by at least 10 cm / 4 inches. The closer the fabric is positioned to the paint, the better. In high RF situations, more folds in the fabric or double layering will increase its effectiveness.

Coverage – How much shielding paint should you order?

T98 shielding paint, comes in universal 5 liter / 1.32 US gallon pails, specially made for shipping, and in 1 liter / 0.25 US gallon bottles.

- 1 liter of paint / ¼ US gallon covers one coat of 8 square meters / 86 square feet. These are conservative numbers, which allows a small buffer.

- You need twice as much paint for two coats and three times the amount for three coats, although subsequent coats tend to use a little less than the first.

- After one or two layers, re-evaluate how much you have used. Apply an additional coat if you use considerably less than calculated.

- Consider your surface: Previously unpainted surfaces, such as concrete or drywall, have high absorption and must be painted with quality primer paint (base coat). This will go a long way in reducing the amount of shielding paint required.

- For anyone on a limited budget, the frugal solution is to apply one or two coats, wait a couple of months, and when the budget allows, apply the next coat. Spread your investment this way and start enjoying your T98 protection.

What materials should you purchase for your project?

Carefully calculate the amount of shielding paint you require, and ask your holistic EMF consultant for advice.

- Order your highly conductive, adhesive grounding tape and shielding paint ahead of time, but use it soon after its arrival.

- You might need a quality primer (undercoat) for previously unpainted surfaces and two coats to hide the black shielding paint later. Consider healthier No-VOC or Low-VOC options.

- A special primer might be needed to cover oil paint for walls, window frames, doors, and baseboards.

- Fuzzy, rough surface paint roller(s) (NAP 10 or 12), paint tray, roller handle, as well as a long extension paint pole.

- Disposable paint brushes.

- A non-permeable drop cloth to protect your floor and furniture.

- Masking tape to secure the drop cloth and protect edges you don't want to paint.

- Paint rags.

- Consider the purchase of a disposable painter's overall.

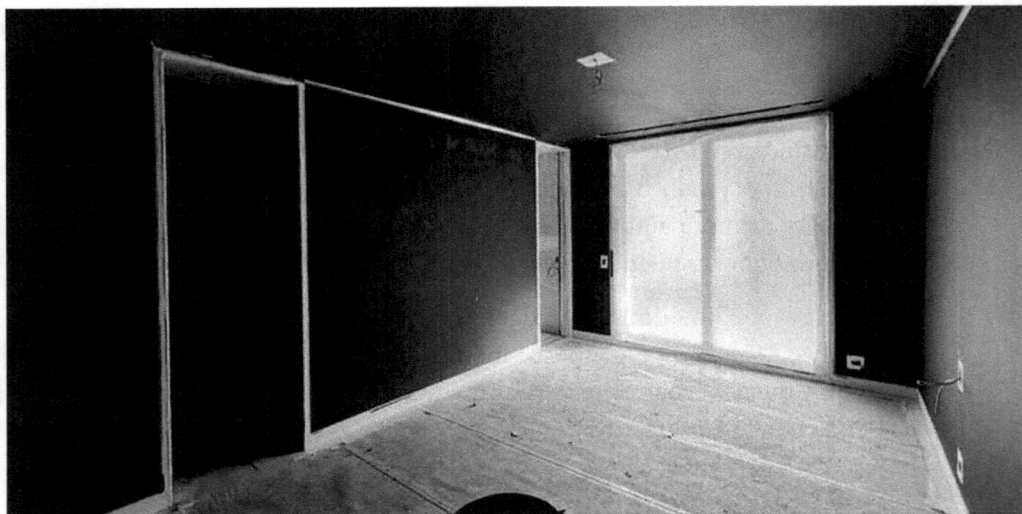
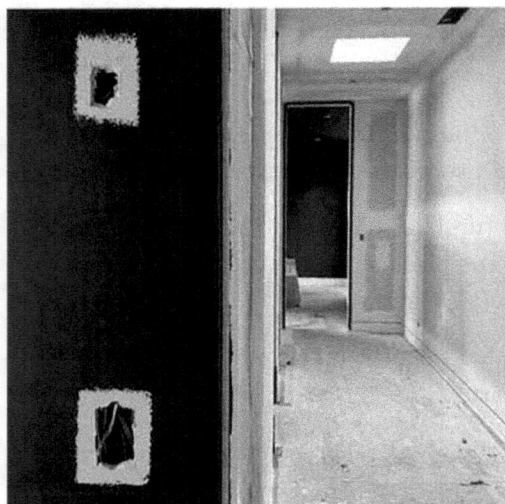
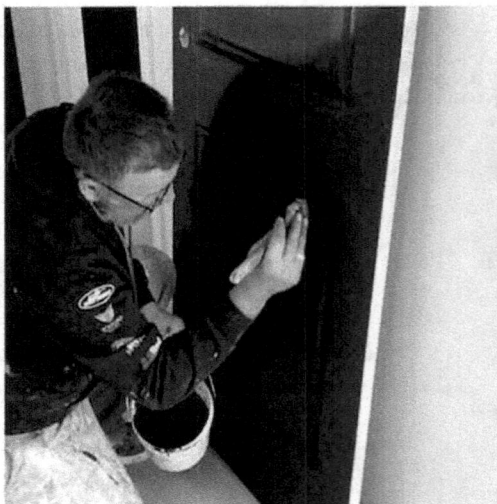
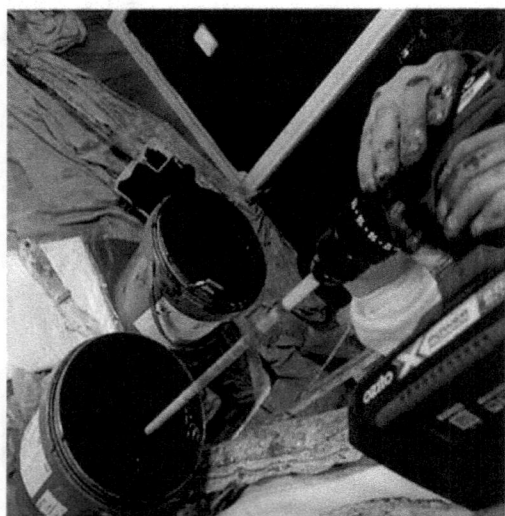
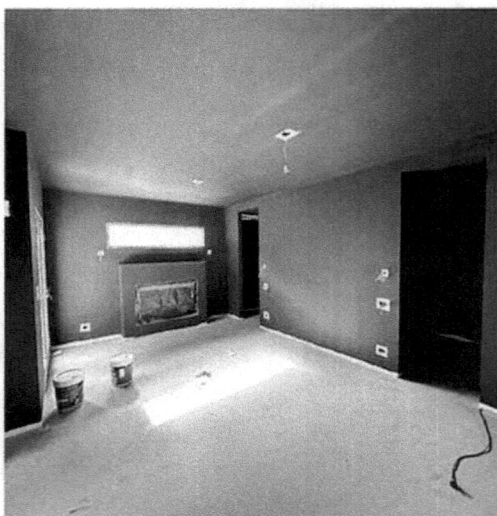

Results after shielding a room

For peace of mind, invite your EMF consultant for a final check. Using your consultant's RF body assessment instruments, you can compare the degree to which the EMF burden on the body is reduced after your shielding efforts. This is also an exciting time for them, as protecting people is why we are in this business.

Even though we enjoy a well-established reputation for successfully helping many families, the level by which the RF will be reduced cannot be guaranteed due to potential variables.

Real-life shielding tests with families

GEOVITAL conducted independent tests on the effectiveness of RF reduction of their T98 shielding paint in real-life scenarios, involving many families who, without previous experience or aid from painters, applied the shielding paint in their homes on their own. The RF shielding results they achieved were phenomenal!

An RF body assessment by your consultant will show if you also achieved such excellent results.

Cell phone signals in a shielded space

Some people expect cell phones not to work inside a shielded space. While this can be the case, a cell phone still might maintain a connection because they will function even with minute signals. This should make us wonder why we need to be exposed to such high levels of RF radiation.

Shielding aims to reduce the RF body values dramatically, and this is typically still the case, even if a cell phone can connect inside the room. It is never a good idea to use a wireless device inside a shielded space, as it will power up to send a signal.

Do I have to keep the door shut?

We have observed many times that when a door is shielded and kept a little open, 10-15cm (4-6 inches), the RF levels on the body remain dramatically reduced. This allows for better ventilation while you can still hear the baby.

Conclusion

Once a proper assessment has been done, you know the facts, and provided your home is not burdened by unfixable magnetic fields from outside, you now have the knowledge to start protecting your home or bedrooms with shielding paint.

Applying shielding paint is an easy way to protect your family from RF radiation exposure now and in the future, giving you peace of mind.

If you found this helpful, please refer your colleagues, friends, and family to this publication as everyone has a right to live in a safe environment.

Enjoy your EMF-protected home!

For more information, please contact me through the QR code or www.radiationfreelife.com

CONNECT WITH ME

Marcus Schluschen
EMF Radiation Specialist, Geobiologist, Activist, Photographer

https://www.radiationfreelife.com

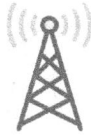

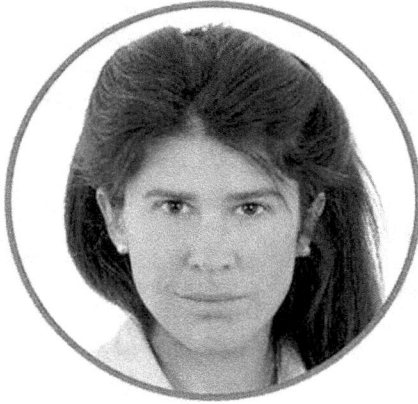

Azul Fernandez

Electrical and Sustainable Energy Engineer,
EMF Radiation Specialist, Entrepreneur

ABOUT THE AUTHOR:
AZUL FERNANDEZ

Azul Fernandez is an electrical engineer based in Northern Italy and is the director of Humankind Wellbeing Engineering, a venture dedicated to creating healthier living spaces by mitigating man-made electromagnetic fields (EMF). Since 2019, she has been a pioneer in domestic shielding solutions, opening the first shielded showroom in the country. Azul is a recognised authority in Italy with extensive practical experience, participating as a key speaker in public national conferences with other well-known Italian scientists and researchers.

While growing up and completing her studies in Australia, she felt a strong desire to serve humanity and confront environmental challenges. During her Electrical and Sustainable Energy Engineering degree at the prestigious University of Adelaide, she received academic assurance that EMF was harmless, yet she couldn't ignore the mounting scientific evidence hinting at potential health risks.

After graduation, Azul gained years of invaluable experience in electrical project design at a renowned international engineering consulting company. Still, she felt a dissonance between industry design guidelines and her belief in prioritising humankind's wellbeing. For instance, she wondered why installing a switchboard behind someone's bedroom or a medium-voltage substation beside someone's office was accepted.

This dissonance prompted Azul to embark on a non-return educational journey from Australia to Europe, where she immersed herself in geobiology and building biology professional courses across France, Switzerland, Austria, and Germany.

Azul's dedication to creating a healthier way of living, coupled with her technical knowledge, makes her a unique specialist. You can reach out to her via the website, www.hkwengineering.com

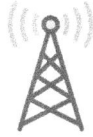

CHAPTER 8

EMF MITIGATION - SHIELDING RADIO- AND LOW-FREQUENCY RADIATION BY OTHER MEANS

By Azul Fernandez

Greetings, esteemed readers and welcome to a journey towards mitigating man-made electronic pollution (EMF) in your home. I am thrilled to embark on this journey as we explore the world of EMF mitigation, discovering strategies to create healthier home environments, with a particular emphasis on sleeping areas. As an engineer and professional EMF consultant, I assess the body for exposure to EMF and the radiation in the air to obtain a clear picture of the indoor EMF burden. Holistic EMF assessments are designed to identify areas in the home where the body may be subjected to unnecessary stress.

There are many ways to reduce EMF radiation in a home, but getting a professional assessment before starting a mitigation project is essential. Most people need the necessary tools or knowledge to assess the house and choose the correct shielding products. Therefore, by understanding the thought process behind a professional EMF mitigation project, the reader will better understand what is needed to mitigate EMF and create a healthier living environment.

In our bedrooms, as with other rooms, we may find three types of EMF radiation that we believe should be eliminated, reduced, or shielded to reduce the burden on the body. These are:

- AC Magnetic fields caused by the flow of current

- AC Electric fields emitted by all standard electrical wires and appliances connected to a live electrical system

- Radio frequency radiation (RF) produced by wireless data transmission, including radio and television broadcasting, telecommunications services, radar and amateur radio.

As we learnt in Chapter 1, EMF pollution is classified as a probable carcinogen, and extensive scientific research has highlighted its adverse effects on human health. Therefore, it is our responsibility to create indoor spaces that promote well-being. The fewer appliances near the bed, the fewer live power outlets and electrical wiring within 2 meters (6 feet) from the bedroom and the less radio frequency pollution inside the home, the more positive and restorative the overnight process. The mitigation of EMF, particularly within the bedroom, promotes a more restful sleep environment, reduces the burden of stress imposed upon the human body while sleeping and may significantly enhance overall well-being.

Mitigating Radio Frequency Electromagnetic Radiation with Solutions other than Shielding Paint

Mitigating radio frequency radiation (RF) in residential spaces demands as much attention as addressing low-frequency radiation. While reducing EMF radiation in every room in the house may be necessary, priority is given to mitigating it in the bedroom. Sleep time is a critical regenerative time for the human body, so we aim to reduce the EMF burden on the body, especially while it restores at night.

Reduce and eliminate EMF as much as possible,
but prioritise a perfect mitigation of EMF in the bedroom.

Mitigation Process

While Chapter 3 details the sources of RF radiation, this section focuses on various mitigation strategies to reduce its impact. One way to reduce the negative health impacts of ubiquitous RF radiation may be to avoid, eliminate and shield ourselves from it.

Firstly, avoid their impact first-hand. First-hand impact means avoiding wearing and using devices emitting radio frequency (RF) radiation, such as wireless headsets, mobile phones, watches and rings. These personal gadgets can interfere with our body's electromagnetic intracellular biological work, potentially causing harm.

Eliminating the extensively used RF-emitting electronic devices is the next step in the EMF mitigation process. Turning them off when not in use and using wired alternatives should be preferred whenever feasible. Some ideas to eliminate RF exposure may be:

- Use wired internet connections
- Turn off wireless antennas such as WiFi and Bluetooth when not in use
- Wire up computer accessories
- Prefer calls using a landline corded phone when at home
- Wire RF sources such as gaming consoles, thermostats, sound and security systems

The longer you connect wirelessly, the more radiation you are exposed to. Prioritise wired technology connections.

Mitigating RF radiation from smart power, water and gas meters can be tricky. If an analogue version is unavailable, the radiation emitted by these meters should be monitored by an equipped EMF consultant. Filters and metal housings may be used to shield these radio signals. It is recommended that professional support is sought for this. Scan the QR code at the end of the chapter if you would like my assistance.

When and How to Shield

Shielding becomes necessary when EMF levels persist, failing to meet holistic consultants' guidelines despite eliminating sources. As an experienced EMF consultant, I apply the latest Standard of Building Biology Testing Methods SBM and the GEOVITAL Akademie GmbH guidelines to assess the levels and propose the most appropriate shielding solution.

The underlying shielding method to block the penetration of radio frequency radiation is to create a Faraday Cage using metallised material on every room surface or volume of space requiring mitigation, meaning walls, doors, windows, flooring and ceiling. A range of shielding materials is available, each with varying shielding effectiveness, application, quality and durability. These can be employed in combination to shield a space and may include:

- Shielding meshes
- Shielding paint
- Shielding fabric

Shielding meshes are commonly applied to walls, ceilings, floor surfaces, roofs and facades. Shielding paints may also be applied to walls, ceilings, floors, facades as well as doors. Lastly, shielding fabrics are utilised to make shielded curtains, partitions and canopies.

Several factors must be considered when selecting shielding material, including shielding effectiveness, third-party laboratory testing reports, durability and suitability to the client's health goals. For the primary objective of safeguarding the client's health, it is recommended to use high-quality, third-party tested materials that promote long-term well-being.

We prefer to verify the shielding effectiveness of a shielded space with instrumentation that assesses the body qualitatively for the presence of RF, as, in our experience, it provides a valuable indicator of indoor well-being.

Shielding Paint

For wall, door, ceiling and floor applications, T98 GEOVITAL shielding paint (described in Chapter 7) is often favoured, particularly when working with clients who suffer from Multiple Chemical Sensitivity (MCS) and Electromagnetic hypersensitivity.

Shielding Mesh

Whilst not as high-performing against RF radiation as shielding paint, which I would prioritise, fibreglass shielding mesh is a versatile solution. It can be used under floor coverings, in between wall linings, wall plaster, roofs and ceilings.

The mesh panels are laid with an overlapping of at least 5 centimetres (2 inches). When grounded, the shielding mesh can also be used as an effective barrier against electric fields, as detailed in the following section. Different grounding options and considerations are available, including electrically conductive strapping or bare wire woven through mesh panels, but a licensed electrician should always connect and verify the connection.

Shielding Fabric

Windows must also be shielded to adequately shield a room against RF. Shielding fabric is thus used to create wave or panel curtains. When RF exposure is high, it may be necessary to make the curtains fuller or add a second or third layer, which significantly increases shielding effectiveness.

When the client resides in a rental property or needs to expedite the shielding process, a shielded canopy may be a flexible option. A shielded canopy is typically cube-shaped, with shielding fabric surrounding all sides and the top of the bed. It may have two side-access openings with an overlapping of at least 30 centimetres (11.8 inches). This overlapping prevents bedcovers from pushing the fabric outwards and opening the entrance. Shielding is completed when the floor, enclosed by the canopy and underneath the bed, is shielded with shielding fabric or a shielding mesh placed under another form of protective material, such as a rug.

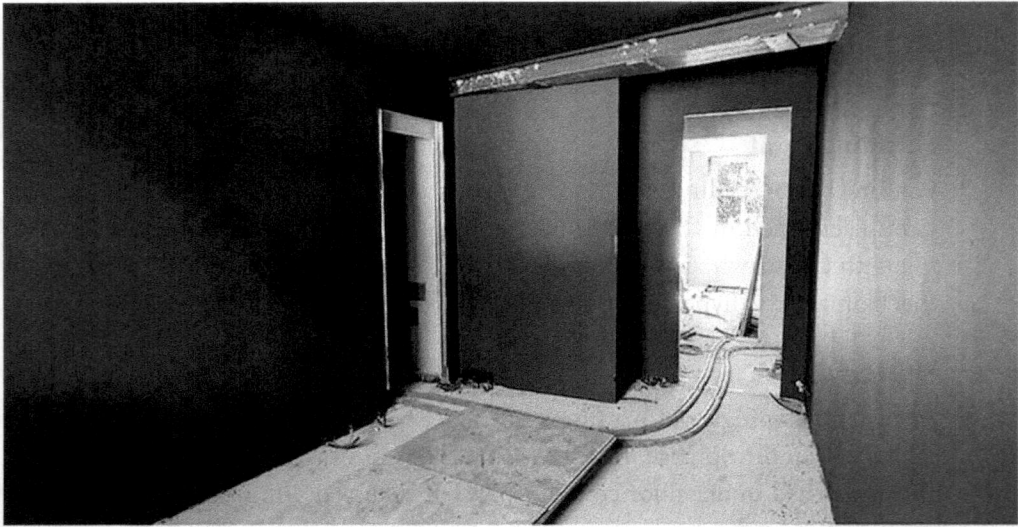
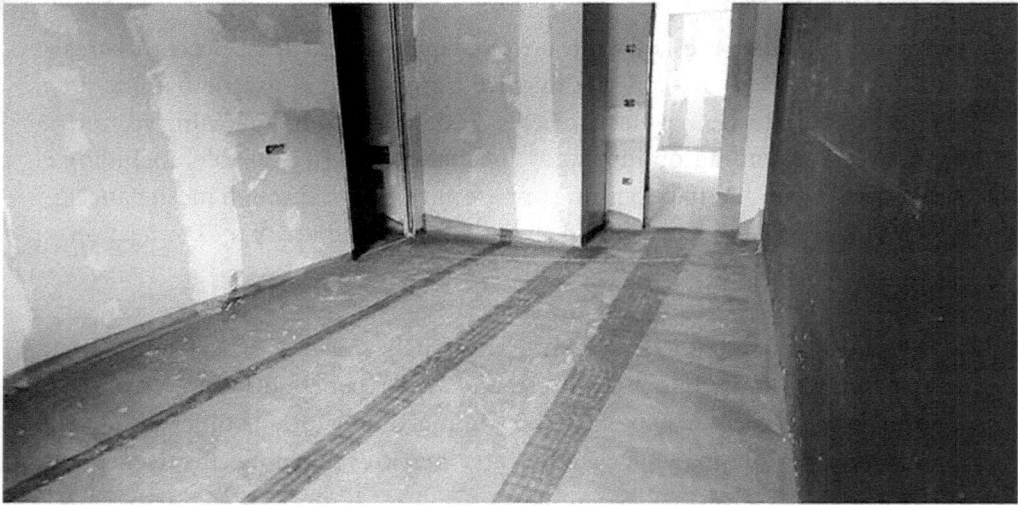
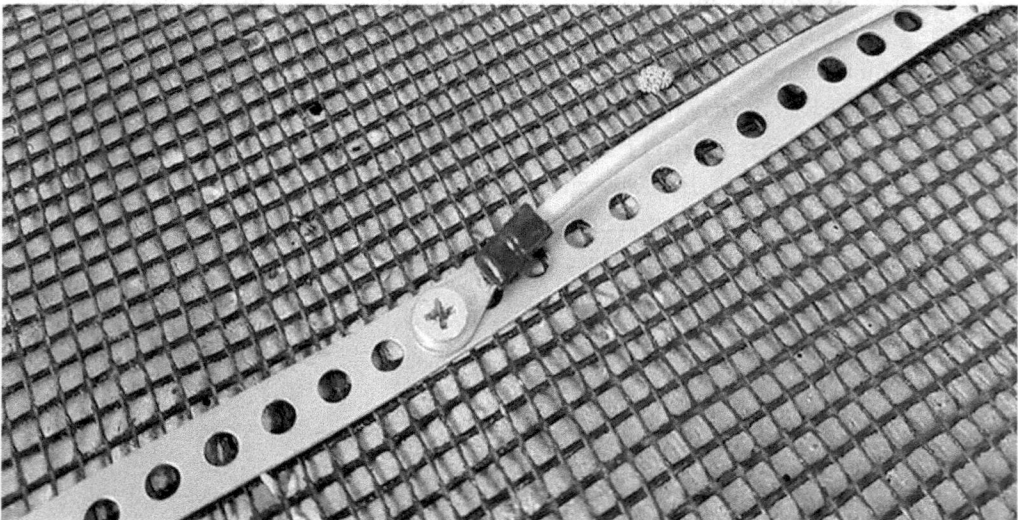

Ideally, the canopy should touch the floor, thereby enhancing the overall shielding effectiveness assessed inside. With ground-floor bedrooms and with no chance for RF penetrating from underneath, the shielding of the floor can often be ignored unless there are electric field anomalies described in the AC Electric Field section. As with other mitigation projects, we recommend professional assistance in selecting and properly installing the shielded canopy.

Light penetration and air permeability of a canopy are additional factors to consider. During warmer nights, it may be necessary to lift the corners to allow air to circulate. We believe that sleeping with the canopy slightly open for a few nights or weeks will not compromise the positive effect of sleeping the rest of the year in an area completely shielded.

The NOVA shielding fabric is often a popular choice for our mitigation projects. Depending on the project's specific requirements, we often use it in combination with high-performance shielding paint or as a stand-alone canopy. This shielding fabric comprises silver-plated copper threads protected by a water-resistant coating and cocooned in either polyester or cotton. Thread coating prevents corrosion and does not compromise shielding effectiveness after washing. Due to the thread coating and polyester or cotton cocooning, NOVA fabric cannot be grounded and additional techniques are required to eliminate AC electric fields.

Shielding a Small Bedroom Space from RF radiation

The following mitigation method is proposed as an alternative to more comprehensive RF shielding strategies. This method is particularly useful for large rooms or teenage rooms where mobile phone usage is often considered 'indispensable'. The method involves shielding a single corner of the room using shielding paint, for example, on two walls and a section of the ceiling. Shielding mesh is then placed under the bed and the remaining sides are covered with shielding fabric to close the shielded volume. It is important to note that wireless devices should not be used in a shielded space. Although it is not ideal for teenagers to overuse mobile phones, this alternative mitigation method should allow teenagers to use their mobile phones in the unshielded part of the room and still benefit from sleeping in a shielded space.

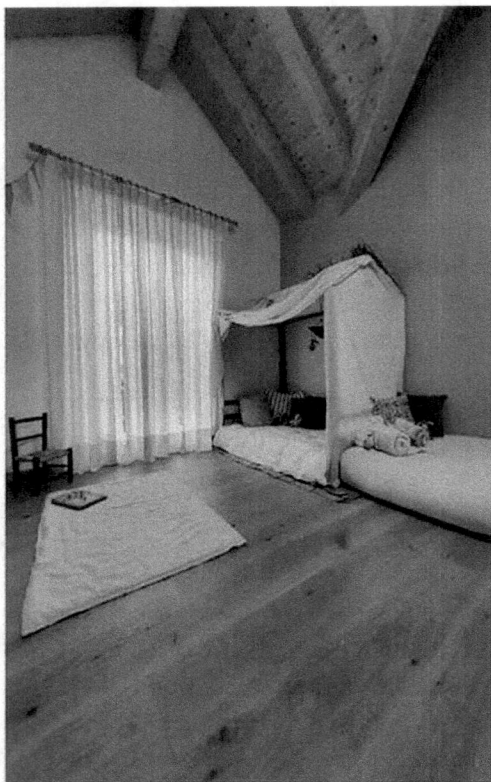

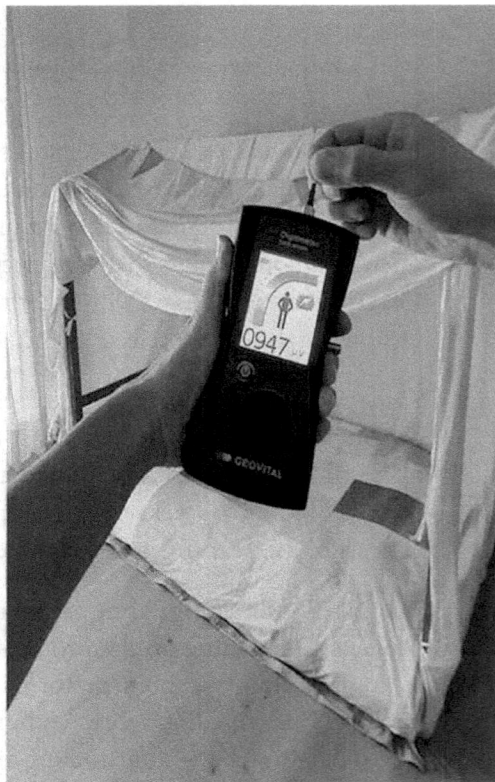

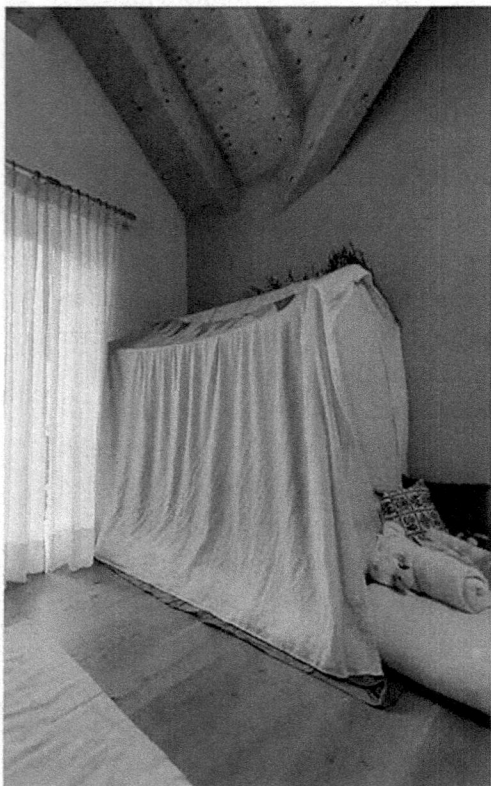

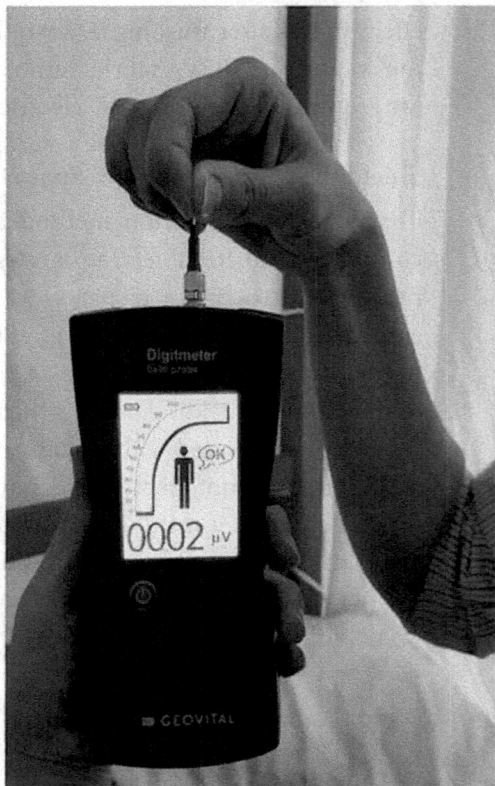

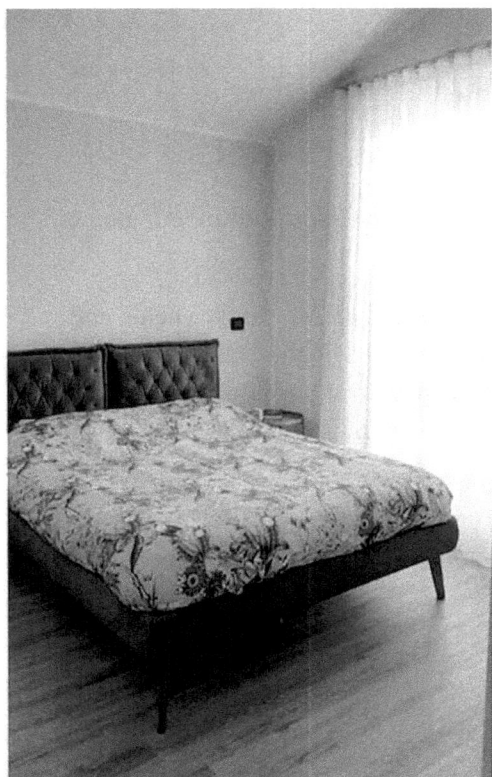

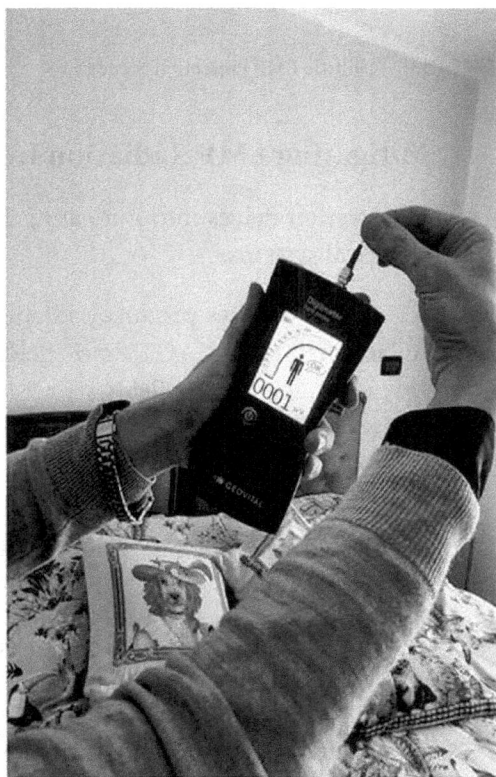

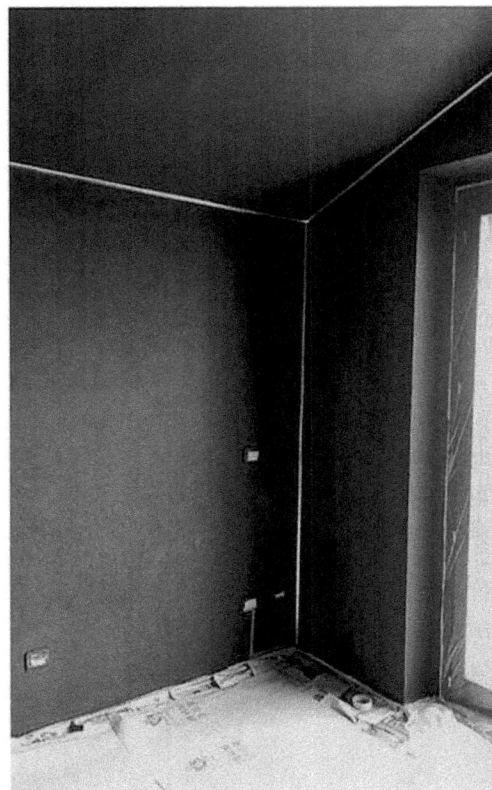

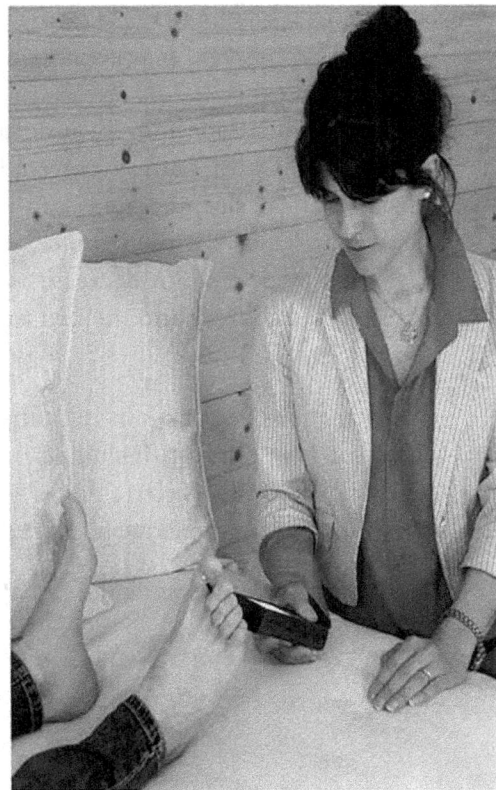

Mitigating EMF Radiation from Electrical Sources

This section delves into mitigating EMF radiation produced by our home electrical systems.

AC power supplies produce radiation composed of AC electric fields and AC magnetic fields. AC Electric fields are produced by the presence of voltage, and AC magnetic fields are created by the current or flow of electricity in a wire. The sources of these fields are detailed in Chapter 2.

AC Magnetic Field Mitigation

In the context of a bedroom, some common appliances that may generate significant and anomalous levels of magnetic fields are:

- Digital and radio alarm clocks
- Bedside lamps
- Electric blankets and water beds
- Battery chargers
- Appliances on standby mode, such as television sets

Mitigation methods may include unplugging the appliances or substituting them with battery-powered options. Refrigerators or washing machines near sleeping areas can be another source of strong magnetic fields, particularly if their motors run at night. In such cases and since magnetic field strength decreases with distance, increasing the distance between the sources and the bed as far as reasonably possible is an effective mitigation strategy.

The presence of anomalous high magnetic fields can also be attributed to more intricate sources, including power transmission lines, wiring errors and stray currents. Electric power meter banks found in multi-apartment buildings can also generate high magnetic fields.

During an EMF assessment, AC magnetic field levels are evaluated, and if they are anomalous, their sources are investigated. If it is a source within the home, such as wiring errors, then an electrician may be able to mitigate it under the involvement of an EMF consultant. If the source is external to the house, from an uncontrollable source, a thorough assessment is done with long-term logging. If the long-term logging reveals anomalous magnetic fields, it is imperative that the occupants relocate their bedrooms away from the source and carefully assess the potential health hazards of continued residence in the house. Shielding may also be considered, but it is an extremely expensive process requiring advanced technical expertise. Magnetic fields have a high degree of permeability, and leaving a small unshielded opening, such as a window, may compromise desired results.

Low-frequency magnetic field pollution is indeed challenging to mitigate and is best avoided. Our professional experience suggests evaluating the levels of AC magnetic field pollution within a residence before its acquisition or rental. Everyone looking for a home is advised to do a basic assessment with a triaxial magnetic field meter. An amateur meter, however, may have a considerable margin of error. Also, the right equipment and knowledge are required to assess the other types of EMF radiation. Hence, once the ideal home has been identified, it is advised to hire a professional EMF consultant to check the amateur meter findings and provide guidance on a holistic mitigation process of the other common types of EMF found in homes.

AC Electric Field Radiation Mitigation

AC electric fields can be found everywhere in electrified homes, as live wiring is usually installed in walls, ceilings and floors. These fields can spread to other surfaces, thus creating a potentially harmful artificially electrified environment. It is essential to note that plugged-in electrical appliances represent one of the primary sources of electric fields in a room and these fields persist even when the appliances are turned off. It is thus recommended to unplug appliances when they're not in use, especially in frequently occupied areas and bedrooms. During our assessments, we prioritise mitigating electric fields in sleeping areas, where the body repairs and restores itself and should avoid the stress caused by EMF.

DE - Dirty Electricity

An ideal home should have an electrical system designed in alignment with human biology, meaning it should be active only when needed. In my professional opinion, assessing and mitigating not only low-frequency electric fields but also dirty electricity (DE) is crucial. DE is a type of EMF that gets into the home wiring from the mains power supply and can be aggravated by smart meters, domestic electrical appliances, photovoltaic systems, battery charges and motors. DE radiates from wiring and appliances like small radio bases into our rooms. Fortunately, electrical filters installed downstream of the power meter can reduce DE when the electrical system is live.

Cut-off switches

One way to eliminate electric fields and DE simultaneously is to use a cut-off switch for one or more electrical circuits. This dedicated device disconnects the voltage supply when there is no load on the circuit. This eliminates the source of electric fields and DE, being particularly useful at night.

There are different hardware options available:

- Automatic cut-off switches
- Remote-controlled cut-off switches
- Low-voltage relays

NOTE: It is important that the system used cuts both the live/active/hot and neutral terminals.

Automatic cut-off switch

The automatic cut-off switch can be installed inside the switchboard or a junction box. When a load is turned on, the cut-off switch reactivates the phase voltage, allowing the load to consume power. The automatic cut-off switch disconnects the phase and neutral connection once again a few seconds after the load is turned off.

From a safety perspective, automatic switches are ideal as electricity is controlled by turning loads off and on from any point in the house. One disadvantage is that appliances that use a small amount of power may not trigger the cut-off switch and a resistor may need to be installed to increase the load value. Appliances that consume power in standby mode may need to be unplugged, or the sensitivity settings on the automatic switch might need to be altered.

Besides being ideal for bedroom circuits, automatic cut-off switches are suitable for electrical circuits that supply the daytime areas of a home. When no power is used on those, the entire circuit can have its voltage removed, creating a more restful space. This could be difficult to achieve in existing homes as the circuitry for sleeping areas might not be segregated from daytime areas. Oftentimes, it is best to rewire special loads like the refrigerator separately and install automatic cut-off switches to control the remaining circuits.

Remote-controlled cut-off switches

Remote-controlled cut-off switches that are controlled from the bedroom with a remote control could be a viable option. Remote controls used in this set-up use a lower radio frequency that transmit only when the button on the remote is pressed to activate or deactivate the circuit.

Low-voltage Relays

A low-voltage relay is an electrical switch that uses a low-voltage electrical signal (typically 12V to 48V, but the lower the voltage, the better) to turn on or off one or multiple circuits. For an accessible cut-off of the electricity in a bedroom, a control switch could be placed on either side of the bed and in the corridor or bathroom.

Essential notes on Cut-off Switches

For appliances that require a permanent connection to AC voltage, such as refrigerators, central heating and cooling systems and thermostats, it is best to have a dedicated electrical circuit breaker with shielded electrical cables, especially if the wiring runs near bedrooms.

Standard circuit breakers are not built for everyday manual operation. It may not only be inconvenient to turn them on manually when needed but may pose security risks in case of emergencies. Rather than turning them off manually, it is recommended to use purpose-built cut-off switches instead.

In conducting a comprehensive EMF bedroom assessment (as elaborated in Chapter 5), we might encounter cut-off switches that were installed without prior inspection by an EMF consultant. Such installation could lead to the sleeping person still being exposed to electric fields, as incorrect or insufficient circuits might be connected to the cut-off switches. Identifying the circuits that cause high electric fields in an existing home, where the location of the wiring is unknown, requires expertise and appropriate instrumentation.

Mitigation in New Electrical Systems

When building or renovating a home, it is important to design the electrical system to reduce exposure to EMF as much as possible. EMF reduction can be achieved through careful planning and design considerations, such as selecting wiring configurations, using shielded cables and strategically placing electrical equipment. By doing so, you can promote a healthier living environment.

The aim is to avoid living and sleeping in a potentially harmful, electrified environment.

Electricity should be active only when there is a need to use it.

Shielding against AC Electric Fields with RF Shielding Solutions

Even by turning off all electrical circuits, acceptable levels of electric fields may not be possible. This can happen, for example, when the main supply cable runs through areas that affect the house's bedrooms.

An effective way to deal with this problem is to shield an area or a room with shielding paint or shielding mesh. These products deflect RF radiation and act as a shield when grounded and placed in front of electric field sources. AC electric fields are naturally attracted to ground (zero potential). Even if RF levels are not anomalous, a room could still be shielded with grounded shielding material to mitigate electric fields. RF radiation tends to increase daily, so it might be logical to protect the bedroom from both RF radiation and electric fields.

Time to Ponder

After reading this chapter, I hope you feel empowered to make positive changes in your living environment by mitigating the effects of EMF radiation. The mitigation process and shielding products that have been proposed are those considered during a professionally guided shielding project. Every home is unique and it is rare to encounter a bedroom with non-anomalous levels of EMF, as recommended by the guidelines I employ.

As an experienced engineer and EMF radiation consultant, I have observed several DIY projects creating problems in the home's health, which could have been avoided by seeking the correct guidance. While it may appear simple to undertake an EMF mitigation project, my experience suggests that it is best to rely on professional consultants to achieve results that are aligned with human well-being.

My holistic approach seeks to create healthier living spaces for the human body. Assessing the body's induced voltage and electric field within a particular space is a valid way to categorise the body's EMF exposure level as anomalous or not. Since we aim to ensure that EMF does not burden the body, it is logical to assess the impact on it directly. In my experience, applying the outlined EMF mitigation methods can create living and sleeping areas where occupants genuinely feel healthier.

As someone passionate about the well-being of others, I understand how daunting it can be to deal with EMF mitigation. I have created a Radiation Mitigation Checklist that you can download and print for your personal use. Scan the QR code provided to access the checklist and find other valuable information and self-guided courses on EMF.

I would be delighted to help you evaluate and mitigate EMF in buildings, be they your home, apartment complex, or tourist facility. Your health and well-being are my top priorities, and I am committed to helping you create a healthier indoor environment for yourself and your loved ones.

CONNECT WITH ME

Azul Fernandez
Electrical and Sustainable Energy Engineer,
EMF Radiation Specialist, Entrepreneur

https://hkwengineering.com

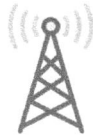

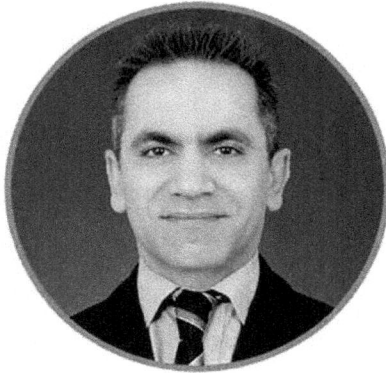

Farzad Nejatpour

Professional Engineer, Master Electrician,
EMF Radiation Specialist, Entrepreneur

ABOUT THE AUTHOR:
FARZAD NEJATPOUR

Farzad Nejatpour is a Licensed Professional Engineer and Master Electrician with over two decades of experience. His company, a reputable electrical contractor with a holistic approach to electrical wiring, is named 'No Radiation Inc.' and is based in Ontario, Canada.

Driven by a lifelong fascination with electrical systems, Farzad's interest began in his youth when he was in grade 6 and got introduced to electronic circuit boards. This passion fueled his academic pursuits, leading him to a strong foundation in Electrical Engineering at university.

In 2017, Farzad's personal life took a turn when his son was diagnosed with Type 1 Diabetes. This event prompted him to delve deeper into the potential health effects of EMF radiation in electrical wiring. His research led him to explore the link between environmental factors and chronic illnesses. After a thorough review and analysis of the radiation assessment and mitigation strategies used by the GEOVITAL Academy for Radiation Protection, Farzad made the decision to expand his expertise with their comprehensive training, turning his personal experience into a professional pursuit.

For many years, Farzad has helped families with a holistic, caring and uniquely complete service to investigate and protect against the risks of EMF radiation exposure. He is uniquely qualified to solve complex EMF radiation issues that an electrician without formal training as EMF consultants is unlikely to understand or mitigate. In addition, Farzad has the specialized equipment to verify that what was fixed has produced the desired results on the body. He also advises families on potential EMF implications for new electrical upgrades and installations.

As a testament to his commitment to children's health, Farzad is available to provide schools with awareness presentations about the responsible use of wireless technology and assist schools that may be worried about EMF radiation exposure or are concerned about constructing buildings in locations close to EMF sources.

Farzad is available for in-person EMF home assessments and support across Canada and provides online assistance to families and electricians anywhere.

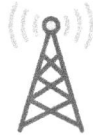

CHAPTER 9

ELECTRICAL SYSTEMS AND ELECTRICAL WIRING ERRORS

By Farzad Nejatpour

Welcome to this chapter on Electrical Systems and Electrical Wiring Errors!

In our modern world, electricity is invisible but essential. It powers our homes, workplaces, and countless devices. But while electricity brings undeniable benefits, there's a growing concern about potential health effects from exposure to non-ionizing radiation generated by electrical wiring.

This chapter will explore two main areas: electrical wiring in homes and magnetic field problems due to wiring errors. I will give a quick rundown on electrical systems in homes and how they work, followed by a little deep dive into how errors in electrical wiring can produce elevated magnetic fields and how to mitigate them briefly.

Electrical Systems

This chapter will provide valuable insights whether you're an experienced electrician, a homeowner, or someone interested in understanding magnetic field exposure.

Electrical terminology can vary around the globe. While the core principles of electricity remain constant, terms used in North America differ from what people are accustomed to in other regions. For clarity, I'll use terms commonly employed by electricians and electrical engineers in the United States and Canada.

In this matter, the term 'hot wire' in North America can be equivalent to 'Live,' 'Active,' or 'Phase' elsewhere and 'GFCI Circuit breakers' in North America are called 'Residual Current Devices' (or RCDs) in other countries. Also, due to the non-combustible nature of building construction materials in European countries and a higher voltage level, which brings down the currents, fewer fires are caused by Electric Arcs, and non-American countries do not use AFCIs.

What is electricity?

Electricity is the flow of electrical charge through conductive materials such as wires. Imagine electricity as water (Electrons) flowing through a riverbed (Conductor). Electricity flows through conductors, powering our devices and lighting up our homes. It can occur naturally, such as in lightning, but can also be generated and controlled for practical use. In our homes, electricity is generated at power plants and distributed through the transmission and distribution lines network.

Generating electricity:

Turbines generate most electricity, which are turned by various energy sources like coal, natural gas, nuclear reactions, or renewable sources like wind or water. These turbines are connected to generators, which convert mechanical energy into electrical energy.

Transmission and Distribution:

Once generated, electricity is sent over long distances through high-voltage transmission lines. These lines carry electricity from power plants to substations closer to where it will be used. At substations, transformers reduce the voltage to a lower level for distribution along local distribution lines. These lower-voltage lines run through neighbourhoods and are reduced through (step-down) transformers to make them ready to be used at the voltage of our electrical devices and appliances in-house.

The Electrical Panel:

Before the electrical panel, a circuit breaker or fuse box, we have an Electrical Meter and service drop outside. Our home's electrical system components start with the electrical panel. The service drop is where electricity from the grid enters our house and is distributed to various circuits through the electrical panel. The electrical panel has circuit breakers or fuses, which are safety devices to prevent electrical overload and short circuits.

Circuits and Wiring:

Electricity flows through our home via a network of wires called Branch Circuits. Each circuit is connected to the electrical panel and powers specific areas or appliances in your home with a certain voltage and current. The wiring is usually made of copper or aluminum because these metals are good conductors of electricity. It's crucial that the wiring is properly insulated to prevent electrical shocks and fires.

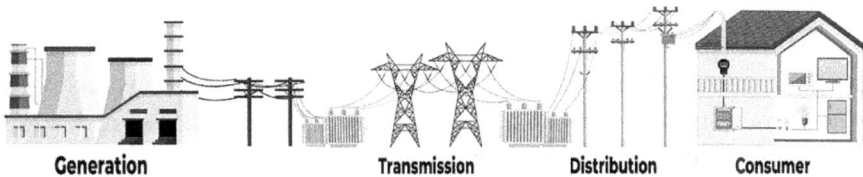

| Generation | Transmission | Distribution | Consumer |

Understanding Voltage, Amperage, and Wattage

Imagine electricity as water flowing through pipes.

Voltage (measured in volts, V)

Voltage is like the pressure pushing the water through the pipes. High voltage is like a strong push, forcing much water through quickly. Low voltage is like a gentle nudge, with less water flowing.

Think of your wall outlet. In North America (US and Canada), a 120-volt system is used; in Europe and most of the world, a 220-240-volt system is used.

Current (measured in amperage, A)

Current is the water flowing through the pipes at a given time. A high current is like a wide pipe allowing much water, while a low current is like a narrow pipe restricting the flow.

Think of the thickness of a wire - thicker wires can handle higher currents without overheating, just like wider pipes can pass more water.

Wattage (measured in watts, W)

Wattage is the amount of work water can do. It depends on pressure (voltage) and flow rate (current). High wattage means the water can do much work, like powering a big machine. Low wattage means less work, like running a small nightlight.

Here's the formula: Watts (W) = Volts (V) x Amps (A).

So, if you have high voltage and current, you get high wattage, like a powerful heater.

These three work together in a circuit like your pipes: The voltage creates the push, the current is the flow, and the wattage is the result - how much work you get out of it. Remember, a safe and efficient electrical system requires balancing these three. That's what electricians are here for: to ensure everything flows smoothly and safely in your home!

Loads:

Load is a general term that indicates any end-user that consumes electricity. It can be a light, space heater, TV, or anything that needs electricity. Loads always dictate how much current must be drawn from the electrical wiring through the circuit. Circuit breakers limit this to safe levels based on the capacity of the wires to carry current.

Power Delivery: Splitting the Current (North America Only)

Another key difference is how utilities distribute power. In North America, we often use a 'split-phase' system. Imagine a single pipe delivering 240 V, then splitting it in half to provide two 120 V circuits to your home. This allows for powering low-power appliances (120 V) and high-power ones (240 V) like dryers and ovens. (3 wire single phase system)

In many other parts of the world, a single 220-240 V circuit delivers power directly. This means manufacturers build appliances to handle higher voltages. (2 wire single phase system)

Grounding:

Grounding is crucial. It's like having a built-in safety valve that prevents electrical mishaps. In case of a problem, the grounding wire provides a safe path for electricity to flow away, protecting us from shock. We will touch on Grounding later in this chapter, as it is often connected to the faults that cause elevated magnetic fields.

Finally, we reach the end users (the load): Our lights, appliances and outlets are connected to the electrical wiring in our walls and ceilings and can be equipped with safety features like Ground-Fault Circuit Interrupters (GFCI), which are called RCD in Non-American countries, or Arc Fault Circuit Interrupters (AFCI). When, for example, you turn on a light switch, it completes the circuit, allowing electricity to flow to the light bulb and illuminate your room. Similarly, when you plug in an appliance, it connects to the circuit and uses electricity.

Understanding GFCI and AFCI Protection in Outlets

Let's talk about the unsung heroes of our home's electrical system: GFCI and AFCI protection. These might sound fancy, but they're just our friendly neighbourhood guardians against electrical hazards.

Think of your electrical system as a highway for electricity. We want the current to flow smoothly from the main panel to outlets and appliances. But sometimes, things can go wrong. That's where GFCI and AFCI come in.

GFCI (Ground Fault Circuit Interrupter): The Shock Stopper

Imagine a leak in a water hose. Electricity can 'leak,' too, and that's what a GFCI watches for. It constantly checks to ensure the amount of electricity going out to an appliance matches the amount coming back. Any imbalance, even a tiny one, could mean a leak – a potential shock hazard. If the GFCI detects this, it acts like a super-fast switch, shutting down the circuit in a fraction of a second. This can prevent a severe shock and can be used to protect us against electrical faults/mistakes that can expose us to high amounts of magnetic field radiation.

GFCI protection is crucial in wet areas like bathrooms, kitchens, laundry rooms, and outside. Anywhere water can meet electricity is a prime spot for a ground fault, so GFCI provides an extra layer of safety.

AFCI (Arc Fault Circuit Interrupter): The Firefighter

Now, picture a spark in your Electrical wiring. This can happen due to loose connections, damaged cords, or a nail in the wall. These sparks, called arc faults, can cause fires. An AFCI is like a fire alarm for your electrical system. It constantly monitors the electrical circuit for these dangerous arcs. Suppose it detects a pattern that suggests a potential fire. In that case, it cuts off the power, preventing an electrical fire from starting.

AFCI protection is critical in bedrooms, living rooms, and other areas where electronics or appliances with cords are present. These are familiar places where loose connections or overloaded circuits occur.

Why do we use both?

They tackle different electrical problems! GFCI stops shocks, while AFCI prevents fires. They work together to provide a comprehensive safety net for our home's electrical system. Sometimes, we can use a combination of AFCI/GFCI breakers or outlets that offer double the protection.

Understanding Magnetic Fields

Electricity flowing through a wire generates a magnetic field. This usually happens when we connect a load to our electrical system. In correctly wired homes, these fields are weak and relatively harmless. However, wiring errors and other factors can create imbalances and significantly increase these fields. Magnetic fields are unaffected by most shielding materials, so it is crucial to identify their source in homes and fix them.

For over 20 years, I've seen it all regarding residential electrical work. Faulty outlets, flickering lights, overloaded circuits, and the occasional mystery-tipped breakers or GFI Receptacles are all part of the job. However, one issue that often goes unnoticed is the presence of excessive magnetic fields in a home. I noticed them years ago when I added a GaussMeter (to measure magnetic fields) to my electrician toolbox. I found out there is more to it than the average electrician thinks.

Now, let's discuss what an electric field is. Imagine a wire carrying electricity like one of those little black plastic pipes you see going through a greenhouse where the water mists out all the way along. The electric field is like the mist coming off the hose—an invisible area of influence around the wire. Unlike magnetic fields, which require current flow, electric fields exist even when appliances are turned off. This means that unlike the magnetic field, which depends on the electricity used for our appliances while they are on, the electric field depends on voltage only. The electric field is there as long as our appliances are connected to electricity. For more on electric fields, see Chapters 2 and 8.

In the average suburb, due to the distribution line being relatively close by, you typically find a low magnetic field level, which is still at acceptable levels. However, 10 to 20 percent of houses have elevated magnetic fields. Every home that has yet to be assessed/mitigated by an EMF radiation consultant has electric field issues.

What can cause a high magnetic field in homes?

About magnetic fields caused by electrical sources inside a home, we can identify the following causes.

-Net current

1. Net Current from Neutral to Neutral Connection
2. Net Current from Neutral to ground bonding in sub-panels or other junction boxes
3. Net Current from 3-way switches wired wrong

4. Net Current from damaged insulators of a cable in electrical wiring caused by drilling, screw, or nail hitting the cable inside the wall or ceiling

5. Net Current from additional current lost by nearby properties tracking through your home

6. Net Current on leaving your home on the connection to the ground because of a broken neutral in the service drop.

-Separation of Hot and neutral

1. Distribution/Transmission lines, especially Single Wire Earth Return (SWER)

2. Knob and tube wiring inside walls and ceilings of older homes

If you suspect excessive magnetic fields in your home from wiring, here's what to do:

Get an Amateur Gauss meter, i.e., TF2, and check if the house's magnetic fields are stronger than outside. Correctly power down your solar system and see if this makes a difference. If you need help, you can go ahead and shut off the main power to the house. If the elevated magnetic field goes away, you may have a magnetic field due to a Net Current caused by an error in your electrical wiring system. But if the magnetic field stays the same, you likely have stray current tracking through your home from other properties that cause a net current in your home.

Call an experienced radiation consultant or electrician. Don't attempt electrical work yourself. An experienced radiation consultant can measure magnetic field levels using specialized meters and identify the source of the problem.

Fixing the Problem: Depending on the cause, solutions might involve fixing a neutral-ground connection, repairing a faulty ground, running a new line, or even replacing outdated knob and tube wiring.

Now let's get back to the sources of Electromagnetic field and explain each one of them in simple words:

What is Net Current?

Each circuit comprises the power source, load, and wires transporting electricity (electrons). Hotwire takes electrons from the power source to the load and neutral electrons from the load to the source (Neutral), and the difference between the current going through the Hotwire and the Neutral wire is zero. Both wires produce a magnetic field in opposite directions, which cancel each other out. The closer the wires are to each other, the more it cancels out. The wires are very close, so there will not be much magnetic field.

In wiring errors, electrons find an alternative return path to the distribution transformer; in this case, the difference between the current on the hot and neutral wires and the magnetic field generated by each do not cancel each other optimally. This will cause a strong magnetic field between the wires with the net current, which can stay strong even with distancing.

Following electrical codes while doing electrical jobs and hiring professional electricians, permits, and inspections can reduce the risk of developing net currents due to wiring errors. The only part of the net current that the electrical code doesn't cover is the heating devices, which produce high amounts of radiation due to high currents and distancing between hot and neutral, which can be avoided by distancing from them.

How can we detect Net Current?

- GFCI Outlets or Breaker (Class A GFCI trips when the current to ground has a value of 5mili-Amps)

- Clamp Amperemeters can detect Net currents if cables are exposed and non-shielded

Gause meters can detect High magnetic fields that are reduced slower Than average with distancing:

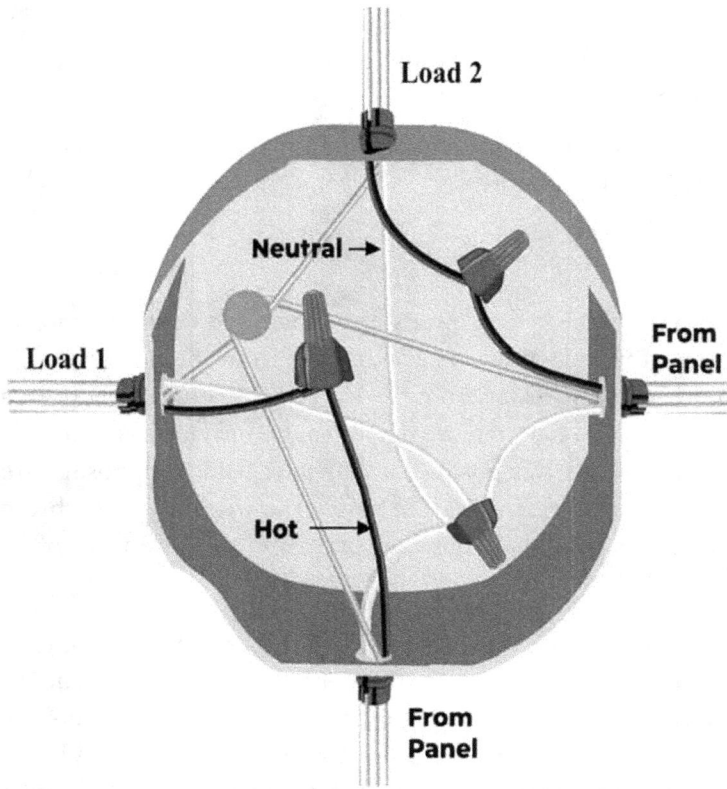

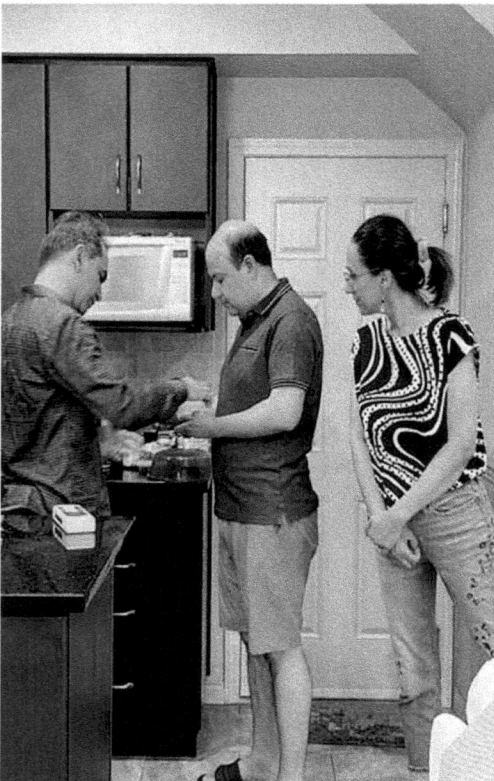

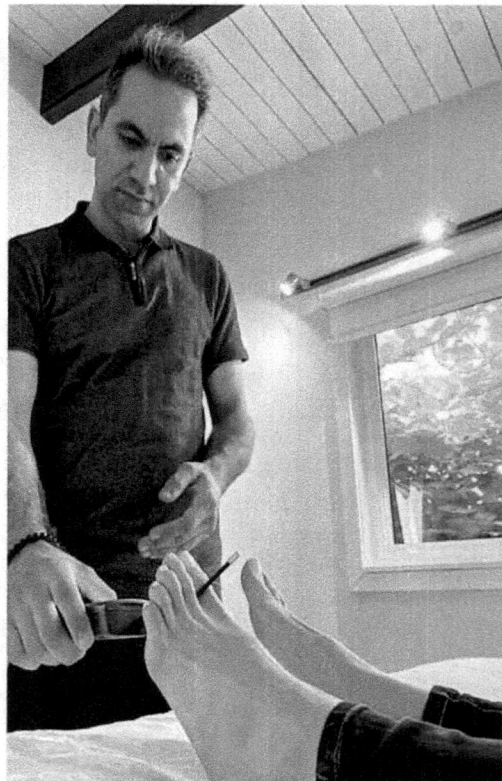

Correctly Wired Subpanel

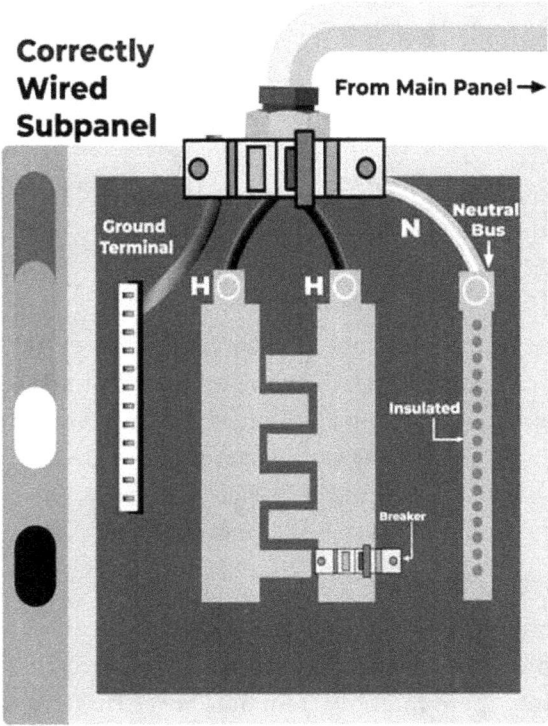

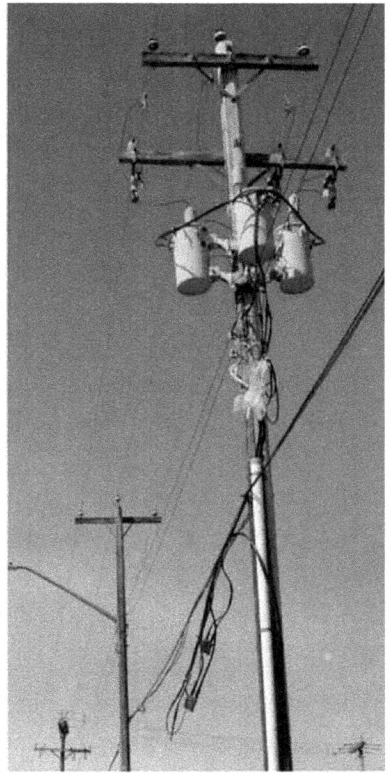

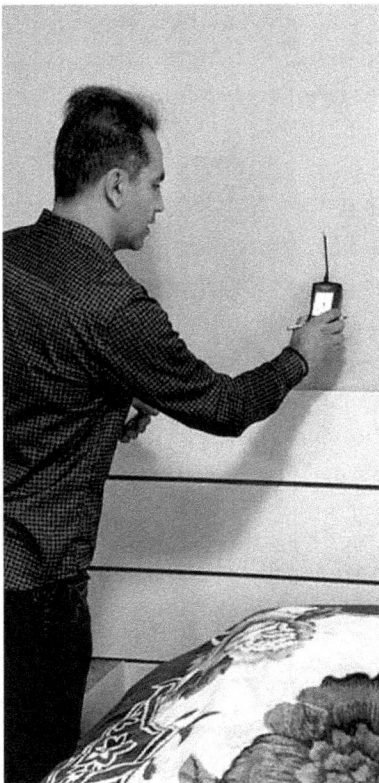

From Main Panel →

Ground Terminal

N   Neutral Bus

H   H

Insulated

Breaker

Incorrectly Wired Subpanel

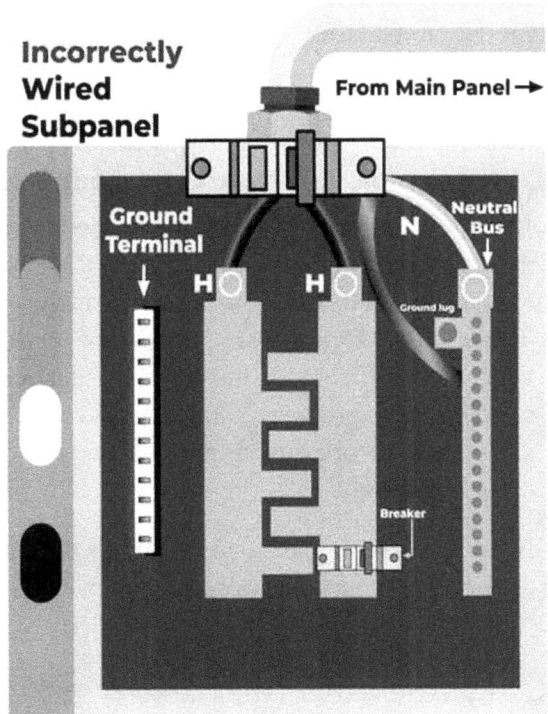

From Main Panel →

Ground Terminal

N   Neutral Bus

H   H

Ground lug

Breaker

- For a balanced (zero net current), the magnetic field is reduced by the square of the distance

- For an Unbalanced (Non-zero net current), the magnetic field is decreased directly with the distance

1) Net Current from Neutral to Neutral Connection

This error usually happens when more than one branch circuit comes to a junction box from the electrical panel. For each cable, we have Hot and neutral; now, for many electricians, connecting all the neutrals in a box is not considered a wiring error. Still, Depending on the country you are in, it may be an obvious code violation and can result in Net Current. While the hot wire is connected to the load, the Neutral has more than one path, returning to the power source.

Finding these mixed-up neutral connections can get tricky, and it may take several hours for a professional Electrician to locate them. In Extreme cases, due to poor workmanship, there might be Junction boxes that are hidden and not accessible (buried inside the wall/ceiling, which makes them untraceable). This is another possible electrical code violation based on the country in which you live. In these cases, disconnecting the contributing lines and wiring for new lines with separate neutral might be an excellent way.

2) Net Current from Neutral to ground bonding in sub-panels

In homes, the neutral is bonded to the ground to offer a path for possible ground faults and to activate protection devices like circuit breakers before energized metal bodies shock/electrocute people or damage equipment. This bond is only on the supply side of the service entry device, which can be a disconnect box or the main compartment of an electrical panel. For all the other sub-panels, neutral buses cannot be bonded to the ground bus as it may be a code violation depending on the country you live in and will cause net current.

It is a very common mistake by DIYers or non-electricians who try to add a Subpanel to their home to add some space for new circuits or avoid running

Correct Basic 3-Way Switch

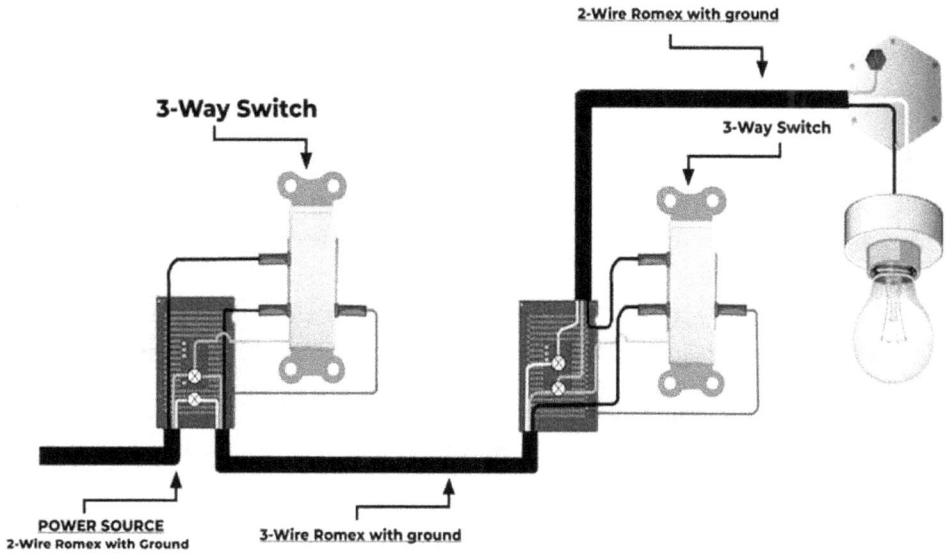

2-Wire Romex with ground

3-Way Switch

3-Way Switch

POWER SOURCE
2-Wire Romex with Ground

3-Wire Romex with ground

Incorrect Basic 3-Way Switch

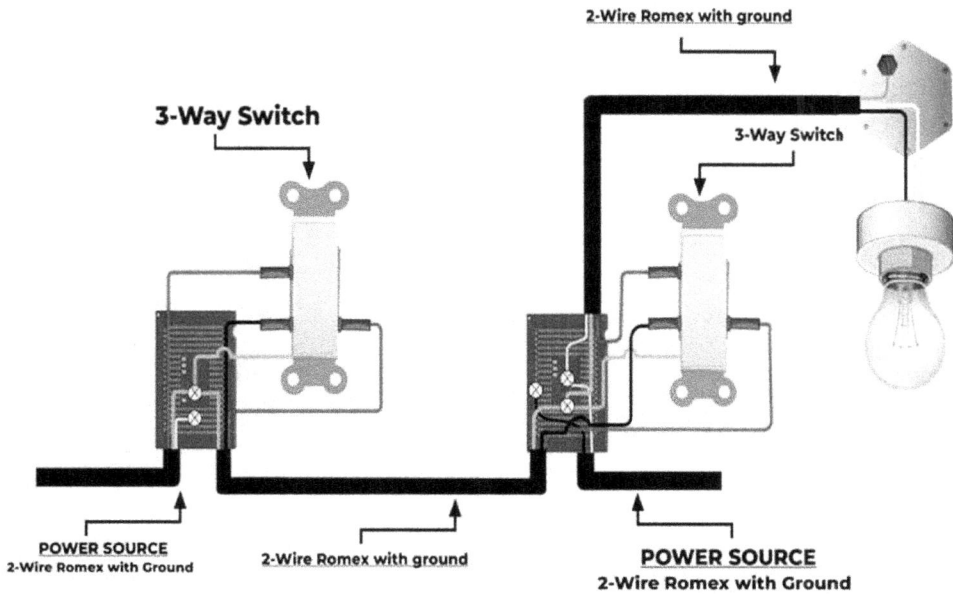

2-Wire Romex with ground

3-Way Switch

3-Way Switch

POWER SOURCE
2-Wire Romex with Ground

2-Wire Romex with ground

POWER SOURCE
2-Wire Romex with Ground

multiple lines for a long distance, Service Rated Electrical panels with Main breakers come with a bonding jumper/screw that connects neutral to the ground terminal if these equipment used as non-service/sub this bonding jumper/screw has to be removed.

3) Net Current from 3-way switches wired wrong

Lights that are controlled from 2 locations are standard in stairs, hallways, or any area with more than one entrance to enable residents to turn on/off the light when they enter the area without passing the dark room, using proper cable/wiring configuration prevents elevated Magnetic field as it allows the light picked up hot and neutral from only one switch, for this configuration a three conductor cable is used between the switches as Traveler.

In old houses/DIY projects, I have seen two conductor cables used to run from the first switch to the next one. An amateur Gauss meter can detect this issue in a house; the good news is, though, we don't necessarily need to run a new 3-wire cable and go through extensive damage to walls and ceiling as there are wireless options available in the market with no damage/extra effort to fix this problem. (they only transmit Radio Frequency when you press the button).

Magnetic field caused by the separation of hot and neutral

As mentioned, the flow of current creates a magnetic field. A hot wire and the neutral have current flowing in opposite directions, and they will make a magnetic field that rotates in opposite directions as well. The magnetic fields will have the same strength when the current is equal. If the wires are close together, there will be a cancelling-out effect. Knowing this, we understand how a net current can produce a strong magnetic field, and in the same way, this explains why we find a stronger magnetic field in any situation where the hot wire and neutral are separated.

Here is a list of situations where the hot wire and neutral are separated, and a stronger magnetic field can be expected:

- Transmission lines
- Above-ground local distribution lines

- Single Wire Earth Return (SWER)

- Solar panel systems, if so, wired

- Knob and Tube wiring

- Electrical panel or near Electrical meter

Creating more distance is the best approach if the problem can't be altered or resolved.

Stray Current - Magnetic field Due to the Grounding to water pipes

Electric Code requires all the metallic water and gas pipes to be bonded to the Neutral/ground Connection at the service entrance device (main disconnect or main breaker panel). This can prevent voltage development on metal bodies of pipes/ducts and Electrical shock as a result of contact of human beings/pets with that.

Metallic water pipes (supply side) have been considered grounding electrodes (metallic water pipes buried at least 600 mm below the finished grade and extending 3 meters). This will create an alternative path for a return to the distribution transformer if there is any issue with the path to neutral in the neighbour's house. Path for return from a neighbour will generate a stray current, which can lead to an elevated magnetic field in the house.

To avoid this, Neutral connections have to be inspected by Licensed Electrical contractors. Any Sign of heat in Connection points can indicate a loose connection in neutral, which needs to be fixed. Also, if the water pipes are isolated, they can eliminate incoming stray currents in our home. In this case, using a Dielectric Union or Replacing part of the incoming water pipe with Pex pipes can Isolate our Electrical wiring from Neighbors and the primary water grid. A separate ground rod has to be installed and connected to the house's Electrical system as per the grounding requirement. A Licensed Electrical Contractor can do this. Also, we still need to restore our ground bonding to metallic water and gas pipes inside the house.

Conclusion

It is not easy to examine the subject of electricity and the causes of magnetic fields in just one chapter. Still, things are more apparent than they were before. We explained the electrical system and its components, followed by a detailed discussion on how internal wiring can produce solid and puzzling magnetic fields. This deeper understanding helps you understand what may be happening in your home or gives electricians an insight into the more profound consequences and causes of net currents and how to address them.

I am based in Toronto, Canada. I am happy to consult with people in Canada and beyond if you want to connect with me. The QR code will take you to my website, where further information can be found and downloaded, and give you a way to communicate with me.

If you found this chapter helpful, please leave a review with your favorite online retailer.

My wish for you is a healthier and worry-free future where YOU are filled with energy!

CONNECT WITH ME

Farzad Nejatpour
Professional Engineer, Master Electrician,
EMF Radiation Specialist, Entrepreneur

https://noradiation.ca

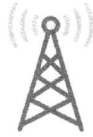

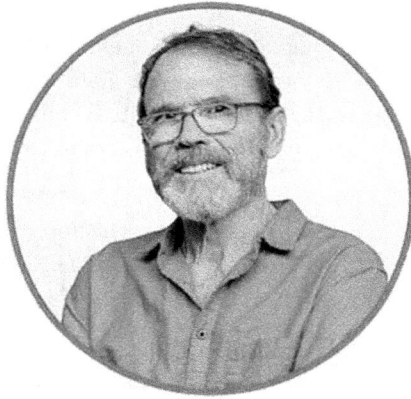

Allen Cheney
EMF Radiation Specialist, Geobiologist

ABOUT THE AUTHOR: ALLEN CHENEY

Allen Cheney is the director of Radiation Prevention Solutions, Australia. He is a former Aircraft Maintenance and Overhaul Engineer with experience in gas turbine engine component overhaul, repair and testing of electronics, avionics, pneumatics and hydraulics. He has been very busy as an EMF Consultant since 2016. He is one of the most well-respected and active EMF radiation consultants on the east coast of Australia, frequently assisting families over an area of 2500km /1,500 miles.

After a healthy farm-style upbringing in Central West, NSW, Australia, then in early adult life in the Aircraft Industry, he faced serious health issues with unexplainable symptoms starting in 2014. He researched and found GEOVITAL and invited one of their EMF consultants to assess his home. This decision would change his life.

During the home radiation assessment, some stresses to radiation were discovered. Sceptical, being a practical-minded engineer, Allen decided to take a leap of faith and implement the recommended solutions—the same solutions Allen now assists other families with.

His health issues, which the doctor had deemed irreversible and were just being managed, started to reduce in severity within months. While the doctor remained fascinated and amazed, this improvement continued and solidified Allen's passion for this field.

Allen is a local and increasingly national authority on verifiably dealing with EMF radiation. He speaks on this subject and has made many enlightening contributions to community focus and discussion groups.

He delivers a detailed and understandable approach to assisting families. He uses GEOVITAL unique professional meters and equipment together with the residents to investigate and understand their situation in actionable detail.

Allen accurately reports, advises appropriate solutions, liaises with contractors to implement advised solutions and then returns to verify results after solutions have been implemented. By going the extra mile, Allen's health clients can see that the health burdens they had in their homes have been dealt with. Allen compares Holistic EMF Protection to getting into a motor car and putting on the protection of a seat belt—you are the safest you can be for the journey—something he wishes for us all.

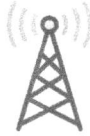

CHAPTER 10

HEALTHIER SOLAR ENERGY SYSTEMS

By Allen Cheney

Welcome to this chapter. I hope you find it helpful when deciding on the installation or health burden mitigation of a solar energy system for your home.

Solar energy in the domestic setting is a relatively new concept that provides a somewhat environmentally friendly option for generating electricity. However, studies reveal that solar energy can have health effects on humans and other living beings. The primary health concern involved with solar energy generation is that people with electro-hypersensitivity (EHS) can get sick from the emitted 'EMF', even in small amounts.

Such health problems may also be triggered by non-native frequencies from cell phones, computers, WiFi and other electronic appliances. The production of solar energy can further aggravate the situation.

Therefore, it is crucial to address these concerns, which will allow better health outcomes for families and the future development of safer solar energy sources that can be utilised by industries and households alike.

A common problem is that modern solar systems use inverters and other electronics. Inverters are designed to transform the solar panel's (PV Array) energy into a consumable form for your home.

Along with most solar electricity supply systems comes the health burden of Electromagnetic Interference (EMI) or 'Dirty Electricity.' It is a Low-Frequency Radio Frequency radiation. Let's call it D.E. in this chapter.

D.E. occurs when the generated electricity exceeds immediate demand, resulting in an inharmonic presence. The following information can help the homeowner discuss the issues with a solar contractor before installing a solar system or considering mitigating an existing system. It can also serve as an introduction to this subject for solar contractors. Spread the word.

People sensitive to the produced radiation may have poor sleep, feel irritable and unsettled, and even experience tingling sensations. Scientists have suggested there are other long-term health effects.

Suppose this information relates to you in any way. In that case, it is best to have a trained expert in this field, with professional equipment, investigate your situation so that you can have an appropriate mitigation strategy at hand. Shielding using various materials is usually the first thing people think of, though it is better to attend to the source whenever possible.

Components

Other than wiring and sub-board/circuit breakers, there are solar panels, batteries, charge controllers, inverters, and converters. I will explain more components and techniques for the system to create or modify a healthier installation.

The solar panels convert sunlight to direct current (DC) electricity. They produce the most electricity when the sun shines directly on them from a clear blue sky. They produce less electricity when cloudy or the sun is lower on the horizon. In constant rain, they produce much less again. At night, they produce no electricity. They commonly produce D.E., which is proportional to the charge or supply rate. Solar panels do not produce any dirty electricity but can radiate if connected to a source of dirty electricity that back-feeds into the solar panel through the wires.

Many solar systems do not have batteries. These systems send any surplus electricity out to the grid. When the house needs more electricity than the solar panels can deliver, it takes the extra electricity from the grid. Some houses have batteries (hybrid) to function during power outages. Other houses are not even connected to the grid at all. The latter is referred to as stand-alone.

An inverter takes the DC electricity produced by solar panels and/or batteries and inverts it to AC electricity that comes out of wall sockets. Inverters work by chopping up the electricity into pulses. This is the case for all types of inverters (sine wave, square wave and modified square wave).

How to eliminate, avoid or mitigate D.E.

Types of inverters

There are several types of inverters used to convert DC to AC, including:

Square Wave Inverter

Generates a square wave output with abrupt transitions between the positive and negative voltages.

Advantages: Simple design, low cost.

Disadvantages: Poor power quality, increased D.E. and inefficient operation of some electrical devices.

Sine Wave Inverter

Generates a waveform that approximates a sine wave, with smoother transitions than a square wave.

Advantages: Improved power quality compared to a square wave inverter and lower cost compared to a pure sine wave inverter.

Disadvantages: It still has inferior power quality compared to a pure sine wave inverter and has increased harmonic distortion.

Pure Sine Wave Inverter

Generates a waveform that is a close representation of a true sine wave.

Advantages: High power quality, efficient operation of all electrical devices, low harmonic distortion.

Disadvantages: More complex and expensive design compared to other types.

Pulse Width Modulation (PWM) Inverter

Uses digital signals to generate an AC output by switching the DC voltage on and off at a high frequency.

Advantages: High power quality, high efficiency, and low harmonic distortion.

Disadvantages: Complex design and higher cost compared to other types.

Micro Inverters

Some solar panels incorporate attached micro-inverters. These are sometimes marketed as AC solar panels. The problem is the micro-inverters, not the solar panel itself. They inherently have 240V AC Electric Fields across the roof where the panels are mounted. In my opinion, the safety of having 240V running across, especially a metal roof, is questionable. See low-frequency electric/magnetic fields in Chapters 2, 7 and 8.

Any kind of wire connected to the system will then act as an antenna radiating the frequencies of the D.E. This is a form of radio frequency radiation. The D.E. can turn home wiring into radiating sources. The key is to find which components cause the problems and provide options for mitigating the existing radiation in your home.

The PV Array

Commonly known as Solar Panels, they generate DC (direct current) while your home uses AC (alternating current). The transition from low-voltage DC to high-voltage AC creates D.E.

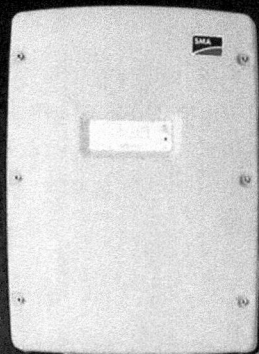

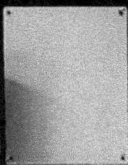

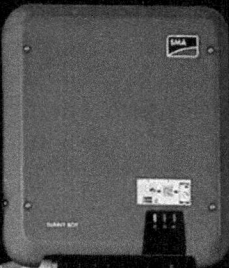

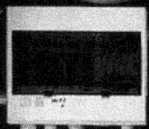

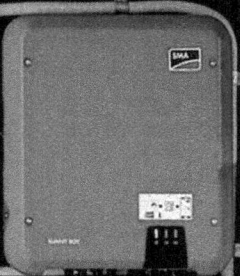

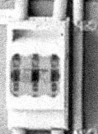

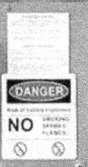

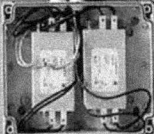

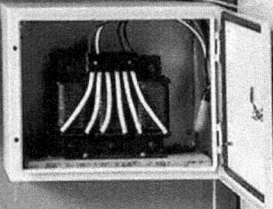

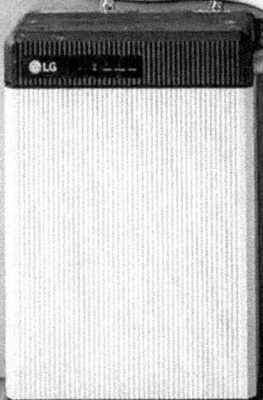

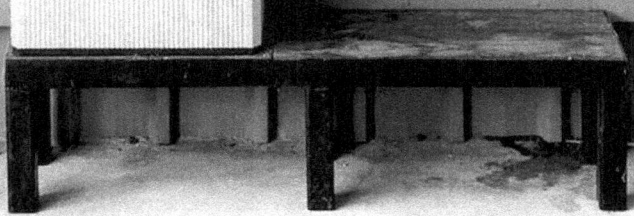

Energy Storage

Battery Types

Solar panels generate electricity during daylight hours but may not generate enough energy to meet the needs of a home during periods of low light or at night. This means homeowners may need to invest in energy storage systems, such as batteries, to ensure they have a reliable energy source when needed.

Lead-acid type batteries

Lead-acid batteries stand out as the best for low-EMF solar systems, as they can use non-pulsing low-EMF charge controllers. However, they may last less time in service.

Lithium-type batteries

Lithium batteries can last much longer. They must use a pulsing charge controller to taper the charging current; otherwise, the battery may overheat and potentially explode. Since pulsing charge controllers produce D.E. it is healthier to avoid lithium batteries. The charge controller turns off the electricity when the battery is full. Otherwise, the battery will eventually be destroyed. This is the case for any battery. The simple charge controllers either allow the full current to the battery or none at all. They do not do any tapering. The more sophisticated charge controllers taper off the current as the battery is getting full. This is more efficient, and for some batteries (lithium especially), it prevents the battery from being damaged. Unfortunately, this tapering is done by pulsing the current thousands of times a second, producing D.E.

Location

Use a separate power shed if possible. One that is not usually occupied during the day. A power shed can house the batteries, charge controller and inverter/s. The solar panels can be mounted on the roof, so keeping the entire solar system away from the house can help. This is a much better setup than trying to mitigate a roof-mounted system with the electronics in a utility cupboard or attached to the living areas or especially places people spend extended lengths of time. The bedroom is the focus as it is the place and time our bodies naturally rest and repair.

Grounding

Grounding the equipment's chassis is good. Grounding should only be done in one place by a licensed electrician, as most countries' electrical codes specify.

It is a common myth that the solution to controlling interference problems is to ground as much as possible and wherever possible. This is a crude way to stop electrical shocks. Some have made mistakes when grounding the negative/neutral wires to various metals around the house, such as metal pipes, steel roofs, steel air ducts, etc. This can cause loops and net current, possibly making things worse.

See magnetic field and net current in Chapters 2 and 9.

Avoiding wire loops

Many solar systems have a wire loop around the solar panels. The positive connector of one solar panel is connected to the negative connector on the next panel, and so on for several panels. This loop can be quite large, perhaps covering nearly the entire roof.

In combination, each solar panel should have its cables (with positive and negative) going to a collection box (string combiner). As the current moves in opposite directions inside a cable, the fields around the wires will have opposite directions too and thus largely cancel each other out. This is why it is so important that they are as close together as possible.

DC-side and AC-side line filters can be installed on the cabling, bringing solar electricity into the house.

The cost can be surprisingly low depending on the issues found and the size of the system. An EMF consultant with practical experience will need to be consulted to choose the correct filter/s for the frequencies to be mitigated.

Low-voltage relays

A preferred alternative, apart from initially installing the advised filters, is a switch that breaks the phase+ wire so current cannot flow on a circuit. However, the neutral wire can still carry D.E. into the household.

Circuit cut-off switches

These are double-poled and disconnect both the phase+ and the neutral/return wires. One or two are typically installed by the door to a bedroom to disconnect all circuits in all the room's walls. Besides blocking dirty electricity, this also eliminates low-frequency electric fields from the targeted circuits.

Any of these options are to be installed by a licensed electrician.

Turning off all the breakers

Doing this will usually eliminate D.E. Be aware that if the system has batteries, they will decline in capacity holding if they are not charged regularly. Breakers are not designed to be used as a switch.

Pure analog DC-only solar

The other rarely chosen option is to use a DC-only system, which was common for off-grid solar houses in the early days before inverters became dominant. Pure DC-only systems are not for everyone, as they come with limitations compared to a typical modern grid-connected or off-grid solar system. With a DC-only system, you cannot sell surplus electricity to the grid, you have to use batteries, and you have to use DC lamps and appliances.

DC is not as convenient as unlimited power from the nearest electrical outlet, although some people with severe electrical hypersensitivity live comfortably with analog DC-only solar systems.

Harmonisers, Balancers, and Neutralisers

If you stop the actual sources of the D.E. (such as the inverter), then the whole system becomes dormant. It is crucial to understand this. If you want to understand the mitigation strategy, avoid trying other ideas that may not bring any improvement.

Many companies provide devices that they claim somehow make EMF harmless. With a vast interest in all things, I have tested various items and found they do not make any difference on any EMF instrument and purchasers are often disappointed or indifferent about their use.

The plug-in to the power point/outlet type capacitors ('D.E. filters') should be avoided. They usually modify the sine wave of the AC from the inverter in a way that could eventually damage the inverter/s.

When the installation is complete

Have your licensed contractor check

A clamp meter on the supply line is used to check the home and ensure there is no net current when electricity is being used. With current flow, a net current presents as magnetic fields from circuits when appliances are in use. Net current in a correctly operating domestic system should be no more than 100mA (milliamps) or 0.1 Amps. See net current in Chapter 9.

Hardwiring the solar system for monitoring

When a solar contractor leaves after installation is complete, they usually leave the wireless monitoring activated even if the owner will not monitor the system.

It is best to ensure the wireless ability is disabled in the Inverter/s. This can usually be performed through the inverter/s brand online portal.

As you are hopefully not using WiFi in your home, go the extra mile and disable the solar system's wireless ability as well.

Monitoring can still be performed by hardwiring the solar system using Cat 6a or better ethernet cabling and network switches, also known as Gigabit switches, which are in turn hardwired to your modem/router. I and many health clients I have helped monitor their solar energy system this way and have not used WiFi for many years. We have successfully monitored the system along with an office which is also hardwired.

The human Alpha brain wave frequency is 7.83Hz, the same as the earth's Schumann resonance of 7.83Hz. (yes, we are designed and constructed by nature) The typical WiFi frequency is 2.4 GHz - 5 GHz (Gigahertz, Giga is billion). These high frequencies were never going to be compatible with human biology.

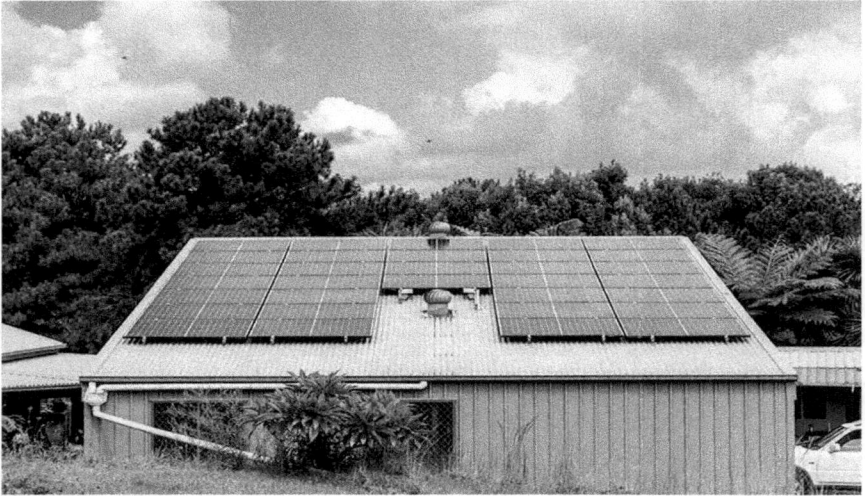

Long-term benefits of using solar power for a home

Cost Savings

By generating their electricity, homeowners who use solar power can reduce their dependence on traditional energy sources, such as the grid, and save money on energy bills over time.

Energy Independence

Solar power systems allow homeowners to generate electricity, making them less dependent on traditional energy sources, such as the grid. This can provide greater energy security, especially in areas where power outages are common.

Increase Property Value

Homes equipped with solar power systems are often seen as more valuable and appealing to potential buyers, which can increase the property's value over time.

Government Incentives

There are government tax credits, rebates, and other incentives available for homeowners who install solar power systems, which can help offset the initial costs of installation and make the technology more accessible.

Some potential long-term drawbacks of using solar power for a home

Initial Costs

Installing a solar energy system can be expensive. This may make it less accessible for some homeowners, especially those on a tight budget.

Maintenance

Solar panels require regular cleaning and maintenance to maintain their efficiency. This may require homeowners to invest time and money into keeping their systems in good working order.

Incompatible with Older Homes

Solar panels may not be suitable for older homes with limited roof space or outdated electrical systems and may require homeowners to make significant upgrades to accommodate the technology.

Interference with Other Technologies

Solar panels may interfere with things like radio or television signals, or cause electromagnetic interference. This may result in performance issues or other problems that can be difficult and expensive to resolve.

Conclusion

There is "no one size fits all" solution to these problems. Going forward, having professional advice from an experienced EMF consultant is ideal.

The issue of dirty electricity and its potential health effects may be new to a solar contractor. New or not, it will probably be received with the same enthusiasm as any company being told their best-selling product, their main income, has a potentially serious flaw.

How much planning or modification is needed? It depends on the situation, the kind of system that is or will be installed, the property layout and the occupants' sensitivity levels.

Before choosing a solar energy system, it is important to carefully consider the costs, benefits, and potential drawbacks of the technology and to work with a licensed and experienced contractor to ensure the quality and safety of your installation.

I trust the subject of creating a solar installation that is less or no burden to health, is a fair bit clearer for you now. In this chapter, I explained the different issues you should consider, enabling you to make more purposeful and informed inquiries with solar power system suppliers.

I assess EMF radiation and Geopathic Stress in homes and workplaces. I am based in Australia and happy to do in-person home radiation assessments with families and video consultations with people anywhere in the world. The situation and available products in other countries may be different. Still, I can likely steer you in the best direction or confirm your planned approach sounds worthy, or that it may have some flaws, in my opinion.

If you found this helpful, please leave a genuine review about this book on the website of your favourite online retailer.

Reach out to me via the link in the QR code and we can schedule an appointment.

CONNECT WITH ME

Allen Cheney
EMF Radiation Specialist, Geobiologist
https://healthstronghold.com/emf-consultant-allen-cheney/?rfs=2

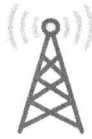

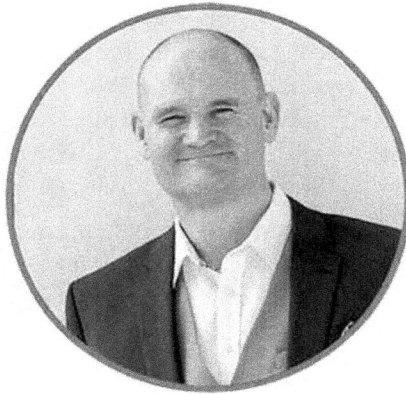

Patrick van der Burght

Radiation-Free Building Specialist, EMF Consultant Trainer
since 2011, International Speaker, Entrepreneur

ABOUT THE AUTHOR:
PATRICK VAN DER BURGHT

Patrick van der Burght, a globally recognised specialist in domestic radiation based in Australia, has been instrumental in transforming the lives of many families. His expertise in assessing and verifiably mitigating EMF exposure from sources like electrical wiring, power supply, phone towers, and more has created many healthier homes. Since 2008, he has travelled the world extensively, assisting ordinary families, corporate high-flyers, celebrities and even royalty.

A family health crisis led Patrick on a fact-finding mission to explore alternative approaches to restoring or protecting health. This is how he discovered the health burden that EMF radiation represents. Triggered by the unfairness of how this affects the unknowing population, he felt compelled to help others.

Patrick has comprehensive international experience with existing residences. He is one of a few consultants worldwide with extensive practical experience assisting architects and builders in planning for and incorporating innovative radiation avoidance and protection measures in new homes, commercial properties and royal residences.

Patrick is an international speaker who has educated the general community and medical professionals. He has been featured in magazines, podcast channels and radio. His educational contributions to the YouTube channel 'Geovital Academy' have over 800,000 views and 46,900 hours of viewing.

Patrick has trained hundreds of people professionally, many of whom now assist families worldwide. His live guided online training program (EMF1) is one of the world's most elaborate, including the possibility to practice under video-call supervision. His in-person workshops (EMF3), held on three continents, have set a new industry standard by enabling students to practice in actual homes.

As Director of GEOVITAL INTERNATIONAL, he coordinates GEOVITAL's availability outside Europe and its English-spoken training globally. GEOVITAL, with its headquarters in the mountains of Austria, has a 40+ year history behind it. Pioneering the development of holistic and verifiable solutions, benchmarked against its clinic's long-term successes with health clients.

Patrick's other business improves the business world through training on ethical persuasion. He enjoys riding his Harley and Scuba Diving. He is happily married and loves spending time with his daughter.

Reach out to Patrick's team via the QR code at the end of his chapters.

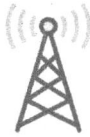

CHAPTER 11

MATTRESSES AND THEIR LINK TO EMF RADIATION AND HEALTH

By Patrick van der Burght

Welcome and congratulations on your interest in this subject. We would be withholding something important from you if we didn't touch on mattresses regarding radiation avoidance and creating a healthy, supportive bedroom. We'll keep this short and tell you what features make sense to demand in your next mattress. Remember that a mattress's recommended maximum life span, if only for hygiene reasons, is 7 to 10 years. How old is yours?

Your mattress is the Missing Link for a Healthier Bedroom

Sleep is the most important time of day when it comes to your body's ability to rest, recover and prepare for the day ahead. EMF radiation interferes with that, but the mattress you sleep on is likely an unexpected burden you must address.

Mattress interactions with radiation in the home

You may never have considered it, but when it comes to EMF radiation, most mattresses worsen your bedroom situation. Water beds and electric blankets are electrically heated and are linked in research to miscarriages and foetal growth defects! [57]

Mattresses with metal springs are very common, but they can also function as big antennas, drawing radio frequency (RF) radiation to you and making the common exposure to electric fields from electrical wiring in the walls and ceiling worse.

Check your mattress with a compass

Many springs in mattresses produce a static magnetic field. Your aim with a bedroom is to create an environment closer to nature. While magnets exist in nature, we did not evolve sleeping on them and this signal is also experienced as a stress signal to the body.

If you'd like to know if your mattress has this problem, grab a compass, notice where the needle is pointing when you are away from the mattress and then place it on the mattress where people would be lying down. If the mattress has a thick foam top, you may need to press the compass in a little, as your body would do. Slide the compass along slowly.

You may find that on many spring-filled mattresses, the needle of your compass starts changing its mind about where north is due to the magnetic fields of the springs. If the needle deviates by more than just 5 degrees, we and other people in our industry would urge you to replace that mattress with one that doesn't do that.

Non-metal filled mattresses are not automatically ok

When it comes to mattresses, the market is very competitive, and the holistic approach to their design is generally not a concern that manufacturers know or think about. Sure, 'health and wellbeing' sells and so does 'back pain', so you will hear of singular features that are aimed at these selling points. Still, manufacturers are oblivious to or don't want to improve other important interactions with the body.

Below, I will list considerations regarding a new mattress, what they could be made from and what it should do for you.

Skin needs to breathe

Your skin is your second breathing organ. If you don't want to seal off 1/3 of your skin surface from oxygen, it would be important to sleep on a mattress with a very open structure to allow air to circulate underneath you. Some mattresses are like plastic bags and in the case of a water bed, that is literally the case. With a relatively simple test, you can get an indication of the breathability of a mattress:

- Put your lips on the mattress. Press down somewhat as your body would.

- Try to exhale (not inhale) a full breath into the mattress.

If it doesn't go in relatively easily, you have your answer. Latex and memory foam mattresses can be particularly poor at this.

Moisture building up in your mattress is disgusting

Everyone sweats during sleep and that sweat goes into your mattress. Good aeration of the mattress material allows that to leave. This moisture is retained in some mattresses with a more closed-cell structure and has trouble getting out. Sweat (which isn't just water) sits there and gets warmed up by you every night. You can imagine how this can become quite an infestation of microorganisms and possibly mould. This is another reason to want a highly breathable mattress.

Subtle incompatibility issues with materials

In complementary medicine, some modalities test for compatibility between food and other materials and the person's body. Examples are kinesiology and electro-acupuncture. When a substance doesn't agree with someone, we refer to that as an intolerance. This can exhaust you during sleep, so you don't wake up with as much energy as you could. As many mattress materials contain worrying chemicals and fire retardants, many produce intolerance reactions in the body. Also, natural materials can cause reactions in many people. Be especially careful with latex, horsehair and memory foam. You can ask a health practitioner of the modalities mentioned above to test what materials bother you and what is neutral.

You should be able to wash your mattress cover

It is easy to have a little accident on a mattress. Sweat, unwanted releases of body fluids, or a cup of tea might make their way onto your mattress. How often have you looked at a mattress without the sheets and thought, 'I wish I could wash that!'. The question is: Why can't you? Mattress covers are stitched into place and become an unhygienic and potentially smelly layer close to your body. You want a mattress where you can easily remove and wash the outer cover.

Where do you get a mattress like that?

The GEOVITAL Academy for Radiation Protection wanted to address the problems related to mattresses by encouraging health clients to buy one without all these problems. Decades ago, they made a checklist and gave it to patients to use while mattress shopping. After some weeks, they all returned, saying no such mattress could be found.

Whilst you could look for a manufacturer who has combined solutions to all these problems with mattresses, the good news is that decades ago, GEOVITAL set out to create a mattress that meets these and more(!) requirements. These mattresses are not readily available in bedding stores because the expectations of high profit margins seem difficult to satisfy with many bedding stores, but natural health practitioners recommend them and the mattress is loved by those who have one.

Made in Austria and shipped worldwide, this mattress is sold under the retail brand PHYSIOLOGA or is available to home assessment clients under the brand GEOVITAL.

"I am very happy with our new Geovital mattress. I had been looking for something like this for a long time and we purchased it without trying it first. I felt the advertising explained the product well and after talking to Patrick at Geovital was convinced that I wanted one of these mattresses! I like a firm mattress and find the Geovital to be supportive yet cushioning at the same time. We are very glad to have purchased this mattress and enjoy a good night's sleep on it." - **Fiona Kelly, Auckland, New Zealand**

Next time you're considering a new mattress for a family member, make sure you get one that works for you and not against you. If you like, you can follow the link in the QR Code for more information about these mattresses.

CONNECT WITH ME

Patrick van der Burght
Radiation-Free Building Specialist, EMF Consultant
Trainer since 2011, International Speaker, Entrepreneur

https://healthstronghold.com/healthier-mattress-information

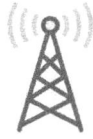

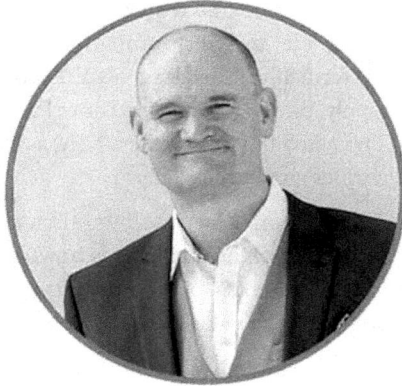

Patrick van der Burght

Radiation-Free Building Specialist, EMF Consultant Trainer
since 2011, International Speaker, Entrepreneur

ABOUT THE AUTHOR:
PATRICK VAN DER BURGHT

Patrick van der Burght, a globally recognised specialist in domestic radiation based in Australia, has been instrumental in transforming the lives of many families. His expertise in assessing and verifiably mitigating EMF exposure from sources like electrical wiring, power supply, phone towers, and more has created many healthier homes. Since 2008, he has travelled the world extensively, assisting ordinary families, corporate high-flyers, celebrities and even royalty.

A family health crisis led Patrick on a fact-finding mission to explore alternative approaches to restoring or protecting health. This is how he discovered the health burden that EMF radiation represents. Triggered by the unfairness of how this affects the unknowing population, he felt compelled to help others.

Patrick has comprehensive international experience with existing residences. He is one of a few consultants worldwide with extensive practical experience assisting architects and builders in planning for and incorporating innovative radiation avoidance and protection measures in new homes, commercial properties and royal residences.

Patrick is an international speaker who has educated the general community and medical professionals. He has been featured in magazines, podcast channels and radio. His educational contributions to the YouTube channel 'Geovital Academy' have over 800,000 views and 46,900 hours of viewing.

Patrick has trained hundreds of people professionally, many of whom now assist families worldwide. His live guided online training program (EMF1) is one of the world's most elaborate, including the possibility to practice under video-call supervision. His in-person workshops (EMF3), held on three continents, have set a new industry standard by enabling students to practice in actual homes.

As Director of GEOVITAL INTERNATIONAL, he coordinates GEOVITAL's availability outside Europe and its English-spoken training globally. GEOVITAL, with its headquarters in the mountains of Austria, has a 40+ year history behind it. Pioneering the development of holistic and verifiable solutions, benchmarked against its clinic's long-term successes with health clients.

Patrick's other business improves the business world through training on ethical persuasion. He enjoys riding his Harley and Scuba Diving. He is happily married and loves spending time with his daughter.

Reach out to Patrick's team via the QR code at the end of his chapters.

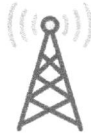

CHAPTER 12

RADIATION-FREE BUILDING

By Patrick van der Burght

Welcome to this chapter and congratulations on your interest in Radiation-Free Building. Building your own home is a privilege and also an opportunity. It is an event you might only do once in your life and you have great expectations about living there when it's all finished. The fact is that most homes are a hub of radiation exposure that bothers our bodies during the day but even more so at night. When you are building your own home, it is the perfect opportunity and most economical time to build a radiation-free^ home.

By making some small changes and small add-ons in the background, you can build a home that not only fits your lifestyle but also supports health.

There is enough research to indicate that low-level non-ionising radiation poses a serious health risk (see Chapter 1). It can impact how we feel, our reproductive potential and how well our bodies can rest, repair and strengthen our immune systems. The cost of building radiation-free and the consultation fees are minor considering the cost of the home, an extension, a tiny house, a free-standing home, an apartment building, a health resort, or a royal residence. Many would agree that keeping you safe in every sense of the word is its primary function.

EMF-free building of a home is not a difficult process, but you need profession-al help in anticipating the various and wide-ranging sources of EMF radiation hidden in your building design, materials and potentially the location. This is where you need an experienced consultant such as myself. Any EMF consultant may offer consultation on this subject, but they rarely have any substantial experience and are hoping to gain some at your expense. For many years, I've trained EMF consultants and trained some of them in radiation-free building practices, but even then, they must continue to involve me on several of their building projects before I can 'sign off' on them doing it all on their own.

Incorporating EMF avoidance and holistic shielding tactics into a home build can seem a bit daunting to tradespeople. This is where a confident explanation and guidance for your architectural and building team comes in handy.

In this book, we work to increase your understanding of the process and considerations of Radiation-Free Building. This helps to pre-plan your project, avoid some exceedingly costly mistakes and may see you make some beneficial design changes early on.

Note: The terms Radiation-Free Building and EMF-Free Building are not to be taken literally. There will always be some radiation left. Radiation-Free Building aims to dramatically reduce exposure to man-made, non-ionising radiation through verifiable holistic solutions.

Why Radiation-Free Building?

Life is precious and so is being in good health. We only have one body and spare parts are in short supply. The human body is amazing. It can deal with many negative influences and will work hard to compensate for the bad things we expose our body to, to maintain homeostasis (balance). The body most definitely has its limits, though, and when it can no longer maintain homeostasis, we start seeing symptoms. That is what a symptom is: the body telling us it can no longer maintain the balance.

As sleep impacts health and recovery so much, we can secure a big win for ourselves and our loved ones by creating an environment where the body is much less or not burdened by man-made radiation. Then there is the discussion of how our reproduction may be affected by exposure to EMF radiation, so in my opinion, all kid's bedrooms should be shielded.

If you are building soon or now, don't miss the opportunity to make a big difference with some prep work, small alterations and additions.

Starting the Processes of Radiation-Free Building

Now is the time to gather information to avoid costly mistakes. Many people organise a 1-hour brainstorming session with me to get my input on their early property plans. This can help to avoid design changes later. Ideally, you should have selected and engaged your radiation-free building consultant before you buy land.

Pick your building team on their willingness to cooperate

Some construction workers are afraid of what they don't know, whilst others are delighted they are about to learn a new skill (which you're paying for) and welcome the inclusions. When it comes to selecting an architect, builder, electrician or even painter, you would be wise to discuss, agree and have something in writing that they will cooperate to include measures to lower exposure to low-level radiation (EMFs) in your new home BEFORE you sign to use them on your project.

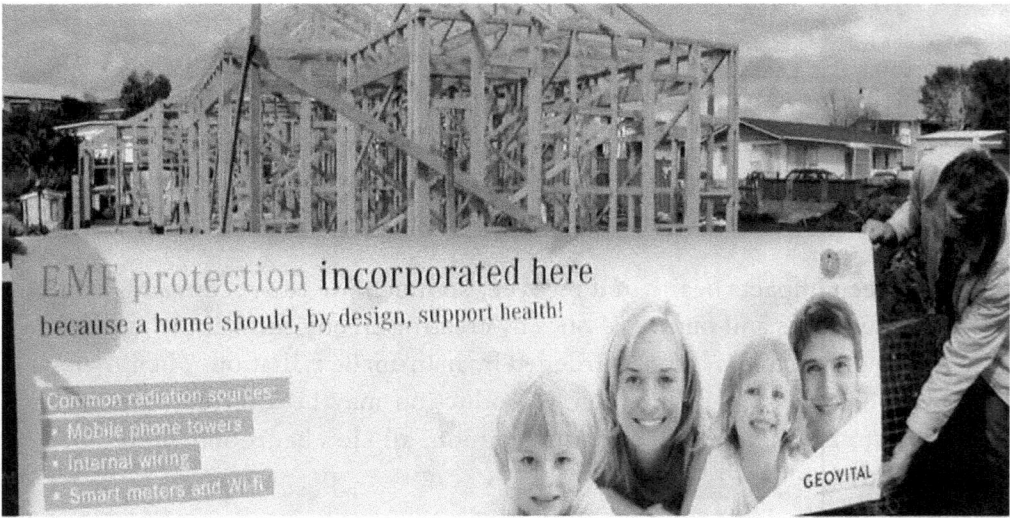

EMF protection incorporated here
because a home should, by design, support health!

Common radiation sources:
- Mobile phone towers
- Internal wiring
- Smart meters and Wi-Fi

GEOVITAL

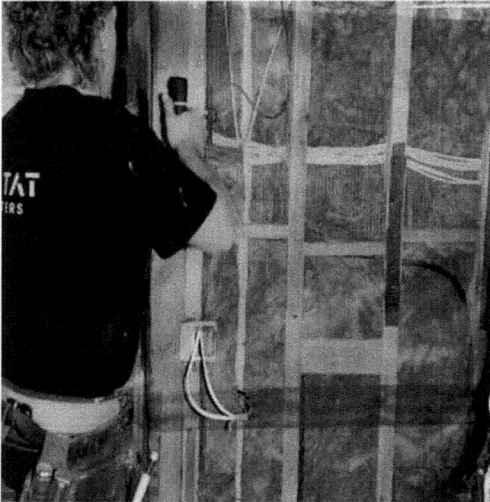

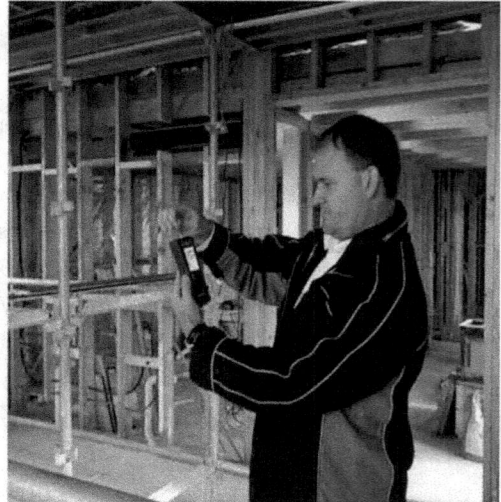

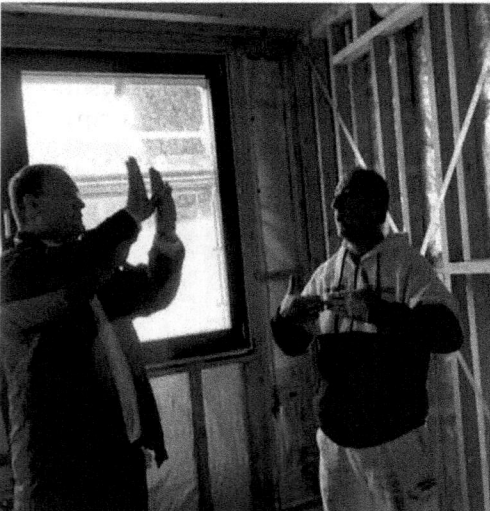

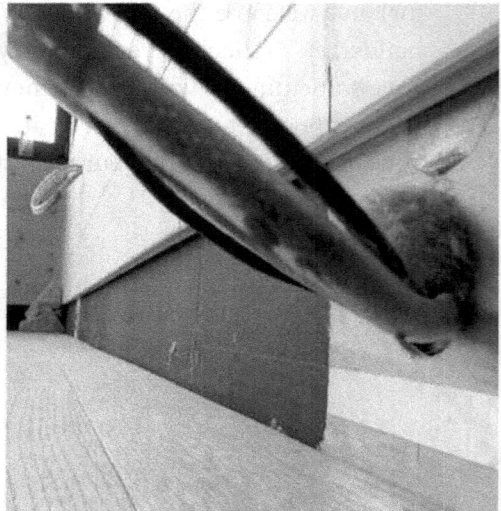

Land Selection and EMF Radiation Avoidance

To figure out if the land you want to purchase or have already purchased is a location you want to stay long-term, some investigation needs to be done. You can do the most important part of this yourself, which is convenient if you are still shopping for a block of land or need to determine where on a block of land it would be wise to build. We are most concerned about magnetic field exposure from nearby transmission lines, local distribution lines (power lines), electrical supply cables (even underground) and transformers.

Magnetic fields can be an unfixable problem on a building site

The flow of electricity produces magnetic field radiation and what you find today may be stronger and larger when power usage increases in the future. Therefore, we should always try to increase the distance between us and power supply cables. Country properties have more space, but be aware of predetermined 'building envelopes' that may limit your ability to place a dwelling.

There are materials you can use to combat magnetic fields, but they are costly, and implementation in homes is, in my experience, only followed by disappointment. Avoiding magnetic field exposure on your new home site should be a high priority.

Chapter 2 explains the sources of magnetic fields and Chapter 4 provides a rundown on how to use a good-quality amateur meter to investigate magnetic fields on a vacant piece of land and what values to avoid! Ideally, you'd have 0.3 milligauss (mG) (=30nT) or less. Somewhere between 0.3 and 1 mG (30 and 100nT), you have to pick a maximum you'll accept, realising it tends to increase over time.

Keep in mind it is not a bad idea to have the site assessed by myself or perhaps one of my consultants around the world under my strict instructions and involvement. This way, using our professional meters, we can make sure your assessment of the situation was correct and investigate for other radiation types whilst we're there.

Not near transmission lines

Transmission lines are predictably bad for us because of magnetic fields in the air, electric fields poring off them like invisible waterfalls and large amounts of current that may be in the ground underneath them and near them. It's best to keep your distance and investigate exposure near them at different times of the day and night.

Electrical power cables nearby

In the city, looking for land with the provision that the local distribution (power) lines are on the opposite side of the street is a good tactic you want to adopt.

There can still be a magnetic field problem when power cables are underground. Therefore, you should have a quality amateur 3-axis Gauss meter in hand so you can investigate and find these underground cables. See Chapter 4.

Radio frequency radiation (RF)

It is always nice to avoid radiation exposure, but our exposure to RF from things like phone towers can increase dramatically when another new tower is erected somewhere. Let's discuss some avoidance strategies.

Not near phone towers

You would hate to buy land only to realise afterwards that phone tower transmitters are nearby. Some transmitters are hidden in fake trees, under manhole covers in the street and in building pillars.

There are websites in various countries where you can find a database of transmitter locations. Of course, new towers are built constantly and more transmitters are added to existing towers, increasing the radiation output.

Many of my clients have homes on properties with beautiful views. When this view is of a city, it often also means that many phone towers will have an uninterrupted line-of-sight view of your home, resulting in higher RF radiation levels in a property.

Note: Professionally, I tie great value to assessing the exposure to RF radiation on the body, rather than assessing the air because the body is a big antenna. Unfortunately, no amateur meters give you this ability at this time. I am somewhat hesitant to encourage you to use an amateur meter to assess the air for RF and base your decisions to shield or not on that input only. When it comes to the air, a level of .005 mW/m² (=5 µW/m²) is considered halfway in the 'slight concern' range. If outside exposure on the ground level is higher than that, either shield or have a consultant come by with a professional meter that assesses the body absorption of RF in that location.

While avoidance is a good idea, most of my radiation-free building clients shield their homes or bedrooms against radio frequency radiation regardless of the RF radiation levels found before the building started, as they always increase.

Building Design and Material Considerations

Normally, I'd like to think I can work with any design clients come up with. Here are a few considerations that may be helpful to you regarding design:

- Avoid placing incoming power cables along the bedrooms.

- Place the smart meter as far away as possible and/or insist on a non-transmitting version.

- Place the circuit breaker panel away from the bedrooms and consider how all wiring fans out from it.

- Metal reinforcement in a concrete slab can be a big problem.

- Electrical floor heating, large appliances like hot water units and air-con systems can produce EMF radiation.

- Glass is more permeable to radio frequency radiation — the more glass you have, the more RF can typically enter.

- Two-story homes get more radiation exposure upstairs.

- More mass in the walls reduces RF exposure. All things being equal, timber frame homes with plaster/gyprock walls will have higher RF than concrete or double brick homes.

- Metal reduces RF radiation, so metal roofs and even wall cladding can help. However, using this alone may not guarantee you get 'good enough' levels inside and you should still consider shielding.

- Solar panels and inverters can be problematic (refer to Chapter 10).

- Data cables should be fitted throughout the home so you can use data wherever you might need it without WiFi (also see Chapter 6).

Regardless of who you end up using as your consultant, you could book a one-hour consultation with me at the very beginning to pick my brain on your project ideas. I could warn you about EMF sources in your design and give you tips on how to protect yourself with the long term in mind.

EMF Protection Solutions

I'd encourage you to incorporate RF protection in your home regardless of today's RF exposure in your location, but please be aware that shielding materials need to be designed with a holistic approach to health, which doesn't seem to be on the priority list of many manufacturers.

Shielding just for the sake of shielding is just not good enough. Just imagine if the product you use reduces RF radiation nicely, but you have intolerance issues with the ingredients used in the product, which affects you slowly over time.

You want to create a health-supportive environment, not just 'less radiation'.

I am proud to say I have always taken this very seriously, and as a result, I've never had any complaints from the families I've assisted over the years. I'm clearly connected with the GEOVITAL Academy for Radiation Protection, but I've always appreciated their concern for material choices as they pioneered and fine-tuned the design of shielding solutions and the most holistic way to assess the situation. They always focused on how this would affect the long-term outcome of the families of their clinic, whom they knew very well.

You may only build a home once in your life.

Your family is worth it to do it right this time.

Shielding Paint

Here, I will keep things 'building'-related so as not to duplicate the information mentioned elsewhere in this guide. Read Chapters 7 and 8 to fully understand what follows.

T98 shielding paint deflects a very large amount of radio frequency radiation (RF). About 15% is absorbed in the paint, which is excellent and most of it is deflected.

You always make a 'box' to protect you from all sides—walls and ceiling. If you shield a room upstairs against RF without shielding the downstairs as well, then you'd have to shield the floor of that room, too. The 'box' can be adjoining bedrooms forming one 'box', or, let's say, an entire home.

Building considerations for the use of shielding paint

T98 shielding paint handles like normal paint but you should consider the following for surfaces that have never been painted before. New walls have a lot of suction. They soak up a lot of the first paint you apply. Good shielding paint is not cheap and it would be, in my opinion, a shame to have it sucked into the wall. Therefore, before you start painting with T98, I recommend you apply a layer of undercoat/primer first.

How many layers?

We used to recommend two layers before we had 5G to deal with and now we see a 3-layer application as the standard. So, for your new home, that is probably also the best approach unless you are far away from civilisation (less shielding may then be ok) or have nearby towers, in which case you want to add more protection.

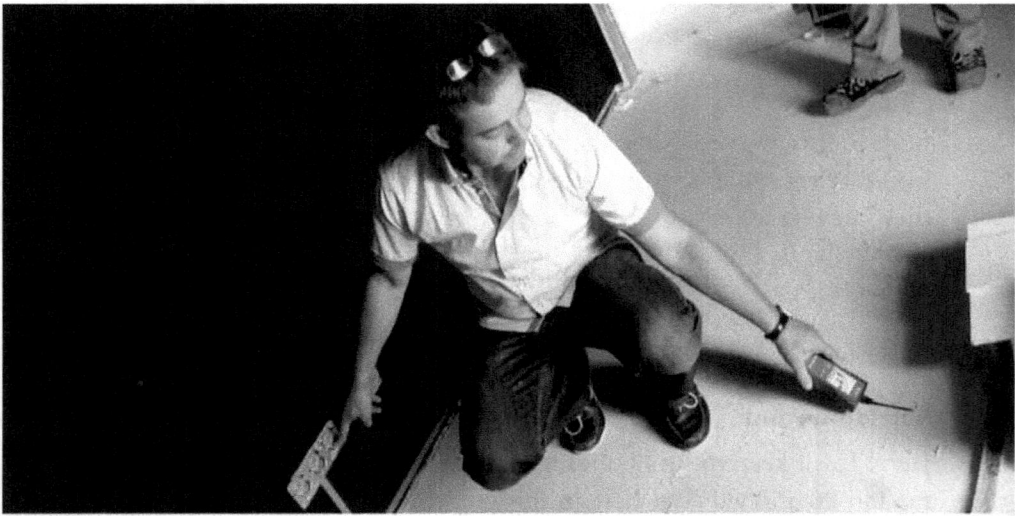
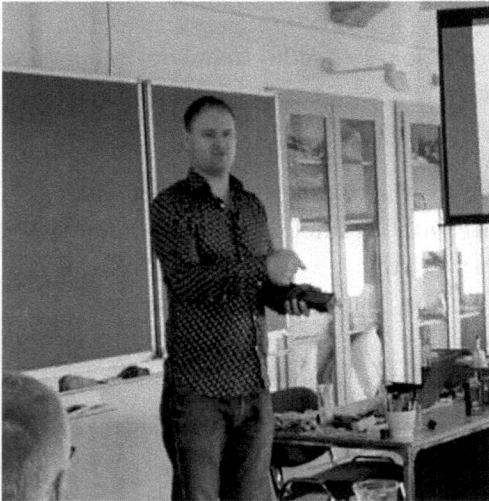
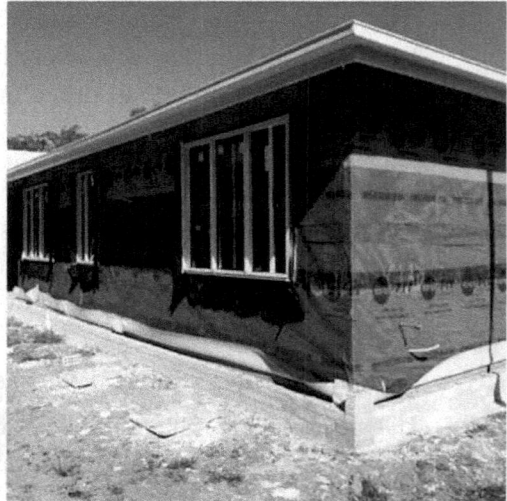
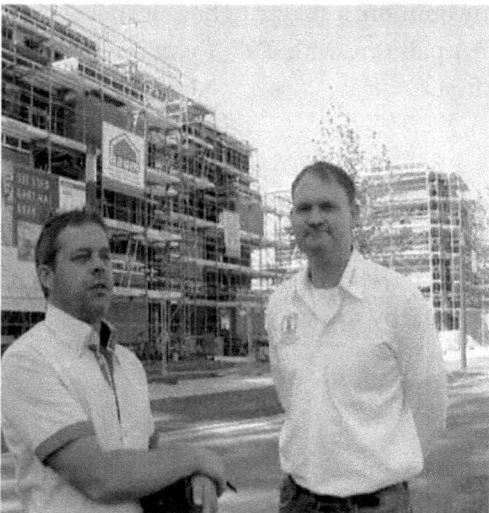
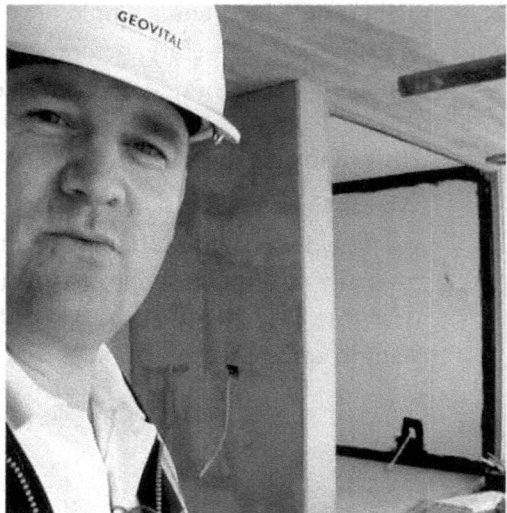

We should consider the future. 6G is already in development and I'm sure 7G will come after. You could consider every layer of T98 as an approximate 7-year barrier. In this analogy, three layers brings your exposure back to how things were 21 years ago. It will offer you the same amount of protection (21 years) 7 years from now. So if our exposure increases, applying an extra 'future proofing layer' would be wise to give you an added 7-year buffer.

Many of my building families apply GPA mesh (discussed later) to the whole outside of the home as a first layer of defence. If you'd do the same, I would normally feel confident to reduce the layers of shielding paint for the inside areas (bedrooms) by one layer.

Regardless of whether you have a metal roof, you need to shield the bedroom ceilings if you're using shielding paint on the walls.

Grounding tape considerations for shielding paint in a new home

Grounding tape use and logic is discussed in Chapter 7. For a newly built home, you may have the opportunity to hide the grounding tape on that part of the wall that will be covered by the skirting boards. It's fine to nail through grounding tape, should it happen.

What do you paint over shielding paint?

We recommend two layers of an undercoat/primer to hide the black T98. After that, you can paint the room in any colour you wish.

Great care was taken to make T98 as healthy as possible. It has nearly zero VOC, which means practically nothing comes out of it after a few days. Putting standard hardware store paints over the top, which are commonly full of chemicals, would be a wasted opportunity. No-VOC and low-VOC paints are easily available nowadays.

GPA Shielding Mesh

Another material I use in homes around the world is GEOVITAL GPA shielding mesh. It is a fibreglass mesh dipped in shielding paint. It has good shielding but not as good as T98 paint. Still, it has its own strengths. I often use it to shield the daytime areas of homes, the floor, and under non-metal roof materials.

GPA can be great behind bathroom, floor and kitchen tiles and other floor coverings. GPA shielding mesh reflects RF radiation; when the strapping is grounded, it forms a barrier for electric fields. If used on the outer side of an external wall, it does not address electric fields properly because the source of the electric fields (wiring) is on the inside of the wall and should be dealt with in other ways.

GPA can be placed nearly anywhere, including on internal walls, so that normal electrical cables can be used in them. It is 1 meter wide (3.3 feet), comes on rolls of 50 meters (54.6 yards) and needs to overlap by 5cm (2 inches). More in Chapter 8.

Shielding fabric

During a consultation, we would discuss the different types of window glass and how this can affect RF permeability. In the bedrooms, though, we often use shielding fabric across the windows as an easy and safe way to close off our protection properly.

NOVA shielding fabric is a silver-plated copper thread coated in a special water protection coating so you can wash it (!) and then cocooned in either polyester or cotton. You can read more about NOVA in Chapter 8.

In a new home, it is often used as (or inside) curtains and partitions. Performance is amazing, but when you have phone towers right outside facing the window, do assume you'll also need to double your NOVA.

Shielded electrical cable

A live electrical cable throws out an electric field that extends about 2 meters (6 feet) from the cable. Using a shielded electrical cable instead removes this electric field exposure.

Shielded cable is significantly thicker and less bendable. It also takes more time to install. The thickness of shielded cable can cause issues where multiple cables need to pass through walls or timber studs.

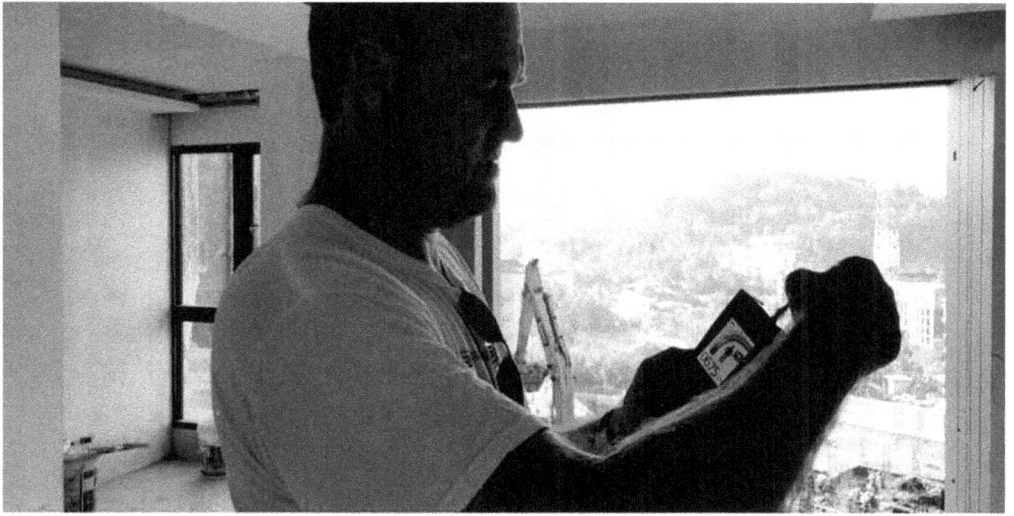

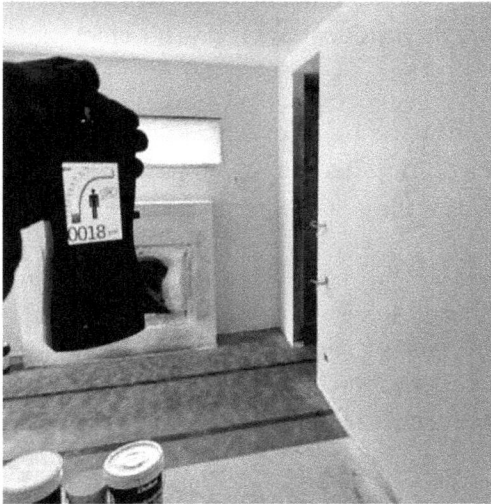

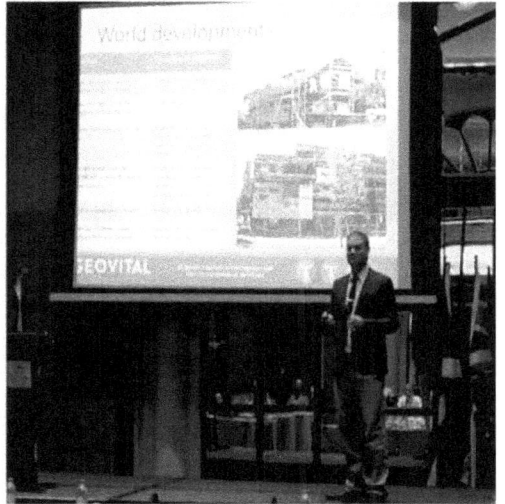

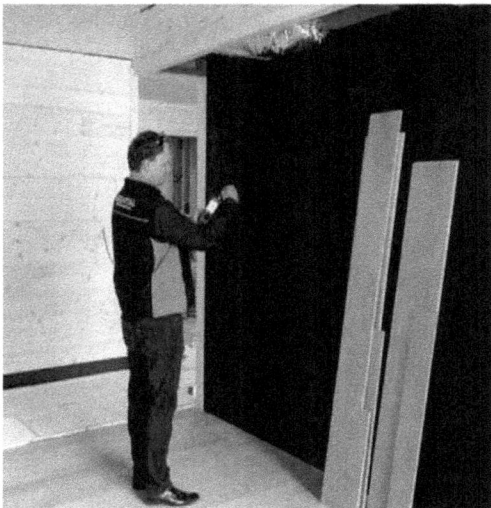

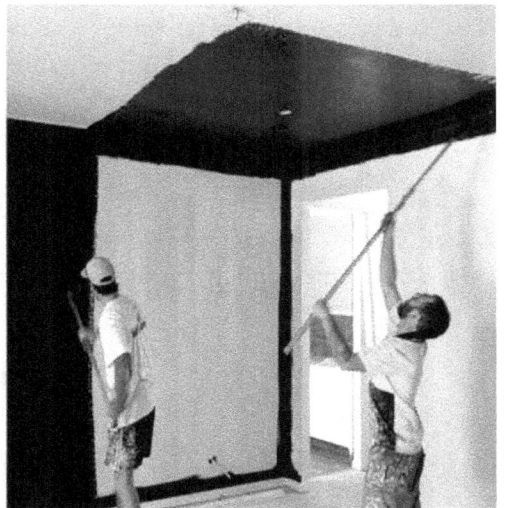

Shielded cable has its uses and can be great in daytime areas that you have chosen not to shield internally with things like shielding paint.

Cut-off switches – Electrical wiring

Electrical cables produce an electric field that extends into the living space. This is not ideal for daytime areas, but especially so in the bedroom, where we need to rest and regenerate. Shielding of the walls and electrical cables can be used to keep this at bay, but appliances you plug in remain a big source of electric fields.

Most people do not want to unplug appliances (bedside lights, bedroom TV) every night, so using automatic or remote-controlled cut-off switches that can remove electricity from the circuit is still something you'd enjoy (see Chapter 8).

To use the switches optimally, careful consideration is given to the design and areas that different electrical circuits service. Bedrooms can have their own circuits and areas that need power constantly can be kept separate.

Enjoy your Healthier Home

Radiation-free home construction is a passion of mine, as it just makes so much sense. My building clients are across the world and I often consult over video call or can fly over to do an on-site assessment or render guidance if desired.

In this chapter, I have explained the need for Radiation-Free Building and covered important steps like avoidance strategies, land selection and some material and design ideas, before eventually discussing EMF protection solutions and some of the specific considerations for building a new home.

Make your building project one that helps your health instead of hindering it. Enjoy it, and if there comes a time you may need to sell your home, it will likely achieve a better price because it has shielding.

If you like, follow the QR code for more information and some valuable downloads. You can also find information on my courses, including the Self-Guided Radiation-Free Building course, the Professional EMF Assessment and Mitigation course, and more.

If you found this chapter/book valuable, please leave an honest review on the website of your favourite online retailer and share it with those you care about.

Good luck with your project. If you are doing a renovation, new home, apartment complex, health resort, or royal residence, I would be delighted to assist you with it.

CONNECT WITH ME

Patrick van der Burght

Radiation-Free Building Specialist, EMF Consultant
Trainer since 2011, International Speaker, Entrepreneur

www.radiationfreebuilding.com

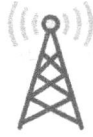

REFERENCES

1. Park, R. (2018b, July 5). Ancient Egyptian headaches: Ichthyo - or electrotherapy?. Pharmacy & Medicine in Ancient Egypt Proceedings of conferences Cairo (2007) & Manchester (2008). https://www.academia.edu/331345/Ancient_Egyptian_Headaches_ichthyo_or_electrotherapy?ri_id=103107

2. Fitzpatrick, R. (2007). Lecture Notes on Electromagnetic Fields. University of Texas at Austin. Electricity. https://farside.ph.utexas.edu/teaching/316/lectures/node12.html

3. Firstenberg, A. (2020). The invisible rainbow: A history of electricity and life. Chelsea Green Publishing. https://www.chelseagreen.com/product/the-invisible-rainbow/

4. Singh, S., & Kapoor, N. (2014, September 23). Health implications of electromagnetic fields, mechanisms of action, and research needs. Advances in Biology. https://www.hindawi.com/journals/ab/2014/198609/

5. Bandara, P., & Carpenter, D. O. (2018). Planetary electromagnetic pollution: It is time to assess its impact. The Lancet Planetary Health, 2(12). https://doi.org/10.1016/s2542-5196(18)30221-3

6. Kay, G. (2023, August 9). Everything we know about Elon Musk's Starlink satellites and future internet plans. Business Insider. https://www.businessinsider.com/elon-musk-starlink-satellites-internet#, SHUNSUKE , T. (2024, January 10). China to launch

26,000 satellites, vying with U.S. for Space Power. Nikkei Asia. https://asia.nikkei.com/Business/Aerospace-Defense-Industries/China-to-launch-26-000-satellites-vying-with-U.S.-for-space-power

7. 2B Group: "There is some evidence that it can cause cancer in humans but at present it is far from conclusive".

    IARC CLASSIFIES RADIOFREQUENCY ELECTROMAGNETIC FIELDS AS POSSIBLY CARCINOGENIC TO HUMANS. (2011, May 31). Retrieved 2024, from https://www.iarc.who.int/wp-content/uploads/2018/07/ pr208_E.pdf.

8. A report providing a Rationale for Biologically-based Public Exposure Standards for Electromagnetic Fields since 2007 and ongoing.

    Sage, C., & Carpenter, D. (Eds.). (2022, June 15). Bioinitiative Report: A rationale for a biologically-based public exposure standard for electromagnetic fields (elf and RF). The BioInitiative Report | A Rationale for a Biologically-based Exposure Standards for Low-Intensity Electromagnetic Radiation. https://bioinitiative.org/

9. RWTH Aachen University. EMF-Portal. (n.d.). Home. Retrieved April 16, 2024, from https://www.emf-portal.org/en

10. Pall, M. (2013, June 23). Electromagnetic fields act via activation of voltage-gated calcium channels to produce beneficial or adverse effects. Journal of cellular and molecular medicine. https://pubmed.ncbi.nlm.nih.gov/23802593/

11. Hosseinabadi, M. B., et al., (2018, December 14). The effect of chronic exposure to extremely low-frequency electromagnetic fields on sleep quality, stress, depression and anxiety. Electromagnetic biology and medicine. https://pubmed.ncbi.nlm.nih.gov/30547710/

12. Sage, C., & Burgio, E. (2018, January). Electromagnetic fields, pulsed radiofrequency radiation, and epigenetics: How wireless technologies may affect childhood development. Child development. https://pubmed.ncbi.nlm.nih.gov/28504324/

13. Johansson, O. (2009, August 16). Disturbance of the immune system by electromagnetic fields-a potentially underlying cause for cellular damage and tissue repair reduction which could lead to disease and impairment. Pathophysiology : the official journal of the International Society for Pathophysiology. https://pubmed.ncbi.nlm.nih.gov/19398310/

14. Gye, M. C., & Park, C. J. (2012, March). Effect of electromagnetic field exposure on the reproductive system. Clinical and experimental reproductive medicine. https://www.ncbi.nlm.nih.gov/pmc/articles/PMC3341445/

15. National Toxicology Program. (2018, November). Cell phone radio frequency radiation. National Institute of Environmental Health Sciences. https://ntp.niehs.nih.gov/whatwestudy/topics/cellphones

16. Falcioni, L., & et al. (2018, March 7). Report of final results regarding brain and heart tumors in Sprague-dawley rats exposed from prenatal life until natural death to mobile phone radiofrequency field representative of a 1.8 ghz GSM base station environmental emission. Environmental Research. https://www.sciencedirect.com/science/article/abs/pii/S0013935118300367

17. Environment Ministry bans mobile tower installation in Core tiger habitats. Communications Today. (2024, February 7). https://www.communicationstoday.co.in/environment-ministry-bans-mobile-tower-installation-in-core-tiger-habitats/

18. Armand, M. (2022, June 8). 4G antenna suspected of disturbing cows will be shut down. Le Monde.fr. https://www.lemonde.fr/en/environment/article/2022/06/08/4g-antenna-suspected-of-disturbing-herd-of-cows-in-haute-loire-to-be-shut-down_5986020_114.html

19. Favre, D., & Johansson, O. (2020, November). (PDF) does enhanced electromagnetic radiation disturb honeybees' behaviour? observations during New Year's Eve 2019. https://www.researchgate.net/publication/346965709_DOES_ENHANCED_ELECTROMAG-

NETIC_RADIATION_DISTURB_HONEYBEES'_BEHAVIOUR_
OBSERVATIONS_DURING_NEW_YEAR'S_EVE_2019

20. Taheri, M., & et al.(2017, January 23). Evaluation of the effect of radio-frequency radiation emitted from Wi-Fi router and mobile phone simulator on the antibacterial susceptibility of pathogenic bacteria listeria monocytogenes and escherichia coli. Dose-response : a publication of International Hormesis Society. https://www.ncbi.nlm.nih.gov/pmc/articles/PMC5298474/

21. 2A Group: "There is strong evidence that it can cause cancer in humans, but at present it is not conclusive" Bortkiewicz, A. (2019). Health effects of radiofrequency electromagnetic fields (RF EMF). Industrial health. https://www.ncbi.nlm.nih.gov/pmc/articles/PMC6685799/

22. Johansson, O., Fragopoulou, A., Grigoriev, Y., Margaritas, L., Morgan, L., Richter, E., & Sage, C. (2017, April 17). Seletun statement. International EMF Alliance. https://www.iemfa.org/seletun-statement/, Home. International Commission on the Biological Effects of Electromagnetic Fields. (2021). https://icbe-emf.org/

23. EMF policy. Public Policy. (2024, April 5). https://www.gsma.com/publicpolicy/emf-and-health/emf-policy

24. AIM, Status & History. ICNIRP. https://www.icnirp.org/en/about-icnirp/aim-status-history/index.html

25. ICNIRP. Guidelines for limiting exposure to electromagnetic fields (100 kHz to 300 GHz). Health Phys 118(00):000–000; 2020. Preprint. DOI: 10.1097/HP.0000000000001210

26. Pall, M. (2018). Response to 2018 ICNIRP Draft Guidelines and Appendices on Limiting Exposure to Time-Varying Electric, Magnetic and Electromagnetic Fields (100 kHz to 300 GHz). https://www.icnirp.org/cms/upload/consultation_upload/Respondent7.

27. National institute of Health, Rome-Italy, 2008. https://www.radiationresearch.org/wp-content/uploads/2018/06/021145_vecchia.pdf

28. The SAR test is inadequate - Environmental Health Trust. Education, Research, and Policy to Reduce Environmental Risks. (2017, July 13). https://ehtrust.org/sar-test-inadequate/

29. Specific absorption rate (SAR) for cell phones: What it means for you. Federal Communications Commission. (2019). https://www.fcc.gov/consumers/guides/specific-absorption-rate-sar-cell-phones-what-it-means-you#:~:text=SAR%20is%20a%20measure%20of,guidelines%20set%20by%20the%20FCC.

30. Belyaev, I., & et al. (2016, September 1). Europaem EMF guideline 2016 for the prevention, diagnosis and treatment of EMF-related health problems and illnesses. Reviews on environmental health. https://pubmed.ncbi.nlm.nih.gov/27454111/ \

31. Final RF charts power density Rev SEP14.XLSX - bioinitiative ... (2022). https://bioinitiative.org/wp-content/uploads/pdfs/BioInitiativeReport-RF-Color-Charts.pdf

32. Natural background levels during normal cosmic activity. Written evidence submitted by Professor Olle Johansson to the UK Parliament in response to MPs inquiry into Broadband and road to 5G, (2020, December 4). https://sb813ca16d3904568.jimcontent.com/download/version/1711094133/module/9476236275/name/Dr.Olle%20Johansson%20%E6%84%8F%E8%A6%8B%E6%9B%B8%EF%BC%88English %EF%BC%89.pdf

33. An academy in Austria recommends that the exposure guidelines should be set, not where harm is demonstrated, but at a lower level to promote the body's self-repair mechanisms. Austria. GEOVITAL Academy. Sulzberg. https://en.geovital.com/

34. International Commission on Non-Ionizing Radiation Protection (ICNIRP) (2010). Guidelines for limiting exposure to time-varying electric and magnetic fields (1 Hz to 100 kHz). Health physics, 99(6), 818–836. https://doi.org/10.1097/HP.0b013e3181f06c86

35. Ahlbom, A., & et al. (2000, September). A pooled analysis of magnetic fields and childhood leukaemia. British journal of cancer. https://pubmed.ncbi.nlm.nih.gov/10944614

36. Grigoriev, Y. (2010). Electromagnetic fields and the public: EMF standards and ... IOP Conference Series: Earth and Environmental Science. https://iopscience.iop.org/article/10.1088/1755-1315/10/1/012003/pdf

37. Spruijt, P., & et al. (2015, January 21). Different roles of electromagnetic field experts when giving policy advice: An expert consultation - environmental health. BioMed Central. https://ehjournal.biomedcentral.com/articles/10.1186/1476-069X-14-7

38. A policy-making principle that allows decision-makers to take precautionary measures to protect from potential harm even if the scientific evidence is not fully established yet.

    The precautionary principle: Definitions, applications and governance: Think tank: European parliament. Think Tank | European Parliament. (2015). https://www.europarl.europa.eu/thinktank/en/document/EPRS_IDA(2015)573876

39. Harremoës, P. (Ed.). (2021, May 12). Late lessons from early warnings: The precautionary principle 1896-2000. European Environment Agency. https://www.eea.europa.eu/publications/environmental_issue_report_2001_22

40. Asbestos. European Environment Agency. (2022, June 27). https://www.eea.europa.eu/publications/environmental-burden-of-cancer/asbestos

41. Biden-Harris Administration finalizes ban on ongoing uses of asbestos to protect people from cancer. (2024, March). Retrieved from https://www.epa.gov/newsreleases/biden-harris-administration-finalizes-ban-ongoing-uses-asbestos-protect-people-cancer#:~:text=WASHINGTON%20E2%80%93%20Today%2C%20March%2018%2C,imported%20to%20the%20United%20States. (The ban allows a transition time up to 12 years)

42. Boice, J., & et al. (2020, August). Evolution of radiation protection for medical workers. The British journal of radiology. https://www.ncbi.nlm.nih.gov/pmc/articles/PMC7446021/

43. Bertová, P. (2022). Europeans for Safe Connections" call for stronger regulation of wireless internet in schools. European Citizens´ Initiative Forum. https://citizens-initiative-forum.europa.eu/blog/europeans-safe-connections-call-stronger-regulation-wireless-internet-schools_en

44. Mobile phones and children. FPS Public Health. (2021, May 17). https://www.health.belgium.be/en/mobile-phones-and-children.

45. Moser, M. (1997, March 1). Evolution of the treatment of hypertension from the 1940s to JNC V. OUP Academic. https://academic.oup.com/ajh/article/10/S1/2S/194309

46. ICD-10-CM Code W90. ICD Codes. (n.d.). https://icd.codes/icd10cm/W900#

47. AAEM. (2021, February 12). Recommendations regarding electromagnetic and radiofrequency exposure. American Academy of Environmental Medicine. https://www.aaemonline.org/recommendations-regarding-electromagnetic-radiofrequency-exposure/

48. Yakymenko, I. (2017, June). (PDF) Nikola Tesla, you and electro-sensitivity. https://www.researchgate.net/publication/319493212_Nikola_Tesla_you_and_electro-sensitivity

49. Carpenter, D. (2015, December 1). The microwave syndrome or electro-hypersensitivity: Historical background. De Gruyter. https://www.degruyter.com/document/doi/10.1515/reveh-2015-0016/html

50. http://news.bbc.co.uk/2/hi/health/2082310.stm

51. Coulon, P., & Rodert , A. (2019, March). Digitalisation – Challenges for Europe - EESC - European Union. https://www.eesc.europa.eu/sites/default/files/files/qe-01-19-295-en-n.pdf

52. Hallberg, Ö., & Oberfeld, G. (2006, February). (PDF) letter to the editor: Will we all become electrosensitive? https://www.researchgate.net/

publication/6836231_Letter_to_the_Editor_Will_We_All_Become_
Electrosensitive

53. Berg-Beckhoff, G., & et al. (2010, November). The views of primary care physicians on health risks from Electromagnetic Fields. Deutsches Arzteblatt international. https://www.ncbi.nlm.nih.gov/pmc/articles/PMC2999946/

54. Environmental medicine officers of the Regional Medical Association's , & Austrian Medical Association . (2012, March 3). Guideline of the Austrian Medical Association for the diagnosis and treatment of EMF- related health problems and illnesses (EMF syndrome). https://magdahavas.com/austrian-emf-guidelines-2012-2/

55. Heuser, G., & Heuser, S. (2017, September 26). Functional Brain MRI in patients complaining of electrohypersensitivity after long term exposure to electromagnetic fields. Reviews on environmental health. https://pubmed.ncbi.nlm.nih.gov/28678737/

56. Belpomme, D., & et al. (2015). Reliable disease biomarkers characterizing and identifying electrohypersensitivity and multiple chemical sensitivity as two etiopathogenic aspects of a unique pathological disorder. Reviews on environmental health. https://pubmed.ncbi.nlm.nih.gov/26613326/

57. Wertheimer, N., and Leeper, E., (1986), Possible effects of electric blankets and heated waterbeds on fetal development, Bioelectromagnetics, 7, 13-22

58. Taheri, M., et al. (2017). Evaluation of the Effect of Radiofrequency Radiation Emitted From Wi-Fi Router and Mobile Phone Simulator on the Antibacterial Susceptibility of Pathogenic Bacteria Listeria monocytogenes and Escherichia coli. https://pubmed.ncbi.nlm.nih.gov/28203122/

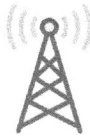

GLOSSARY OF TERMS

BioInitiative Report: A report that summarises research on the health effects of EMFs and provides recommendations for safety standards.

Bluetooth: A wireless technology standard used for exchanging data between fixed and mobile devices over short distances.

Blood-Brain Barrier: A selective permeability barrier that protects the brain from certain substances in the blood that may be harmful.

Dirty Electricity: Electrical pollution that is a form of electromagnetic interference, caused by interruptions in the flow of electrical current.

Electroacupuncture: A form of acupuncture where a small electric current is passed through acupuncture points. Diagnosis depends on measuring the relative electrical conductance and its time dependence.

Electromagnetic Fields (EMFs): Invisible areas of energy, often referred to as radiation, associated with the use of electrical power and various forms of natural and man-made lighting.

Electromagnetic Hypersensitivity (EHS): A condition characterised by various symptoms attributed to exposure to different types of EMF radiation.

GEOVITAL: An educational institution with a history in natural health, specialising in research of health risks associated with EMF exposure, offering home assessments, mitigation solutions and training on those subjects.

Grounding (Earthing): When related to the practice of connecting oneself to the earth, this technique helps to eliminate a static charge that may be present in the body.

High-Frequency Radiation: EMFs that include radio waves, microwaves, and other forms of radiation used in wireless communication.

Ionizing Radiation: Radiation with enough energy to remove tightly bound electrons from atoms, thus creating ions.

Low-Frequency Radiation: EMFs that are typically emitted by electrical appliances, power lines, and other sources that use electric power.

Net Current: A state where the current that moves through a live/active/ hot wire is not equal to the current returning on the associated neutral wire. As the magnetic fields produced by both wires are then unequal, a strong magnetic field will result.

Neurodegenerative Diseases: A range of conditions which primarily affect the neurons in the human brain, such as Alzheimer's disease.

Non-Ionizing Radiation: A type of electromagnetic radiation that does not carry enough energy to ionize atoms or molecules.

Oxidative Stress: An imbalance between free radicals and antioxidants in your body, which can be exacerbated by exposure to EMFs.

Precautionary Principle: A principle that advocates for preventive action in the face of uncertainty, erring on the side of caution to prevent harm when it is within our power to do so, even if some cause and effect relationships are not fully established scientifically.

Radio Frequency (RF) Radiation: A type of non-ionizing radiation that is emitted by various electronic devices and wireless communication technologies, such as cell phones, WiFi, and Bluetooth.

Shielding Fabric: Specially engineered fabric in which finely woven metal threads form a mesh cocooned in a material like polyester or cotton to make a material similar in look and feel to sheer fabric that can reflect radiofrequency radiation. It is typically used as curtaining, partitions or canopies.

Shielding Paint: Specially formulated paint that can reduce exposure to particular types of EMF radiation by reflecting and absorbing this radiation.

Smart Meters: Electronic devices that record energy consumption in homes and businesses and communicate this information to the utility for monitoring and billing, often emitting RF radiation.

Solar Power Systems: Systems that use solar panels to convert sunlight into electricity, which can produce EMF radiation. Also referred to as a photovoltaic (PV) system.

Specific Absorption Rate (SAR): A measure of the rate at which energy is absorbed by the human body when exposed to a radio frequency electromagnetic field.

Voltage-Gated Calcium Channels: Channels in the cell membrane that allow the movement of calcium ions into the cell, which can be affected by EMFs.

WiFi (Wireless Fidelity): A technology that allows electronic devices to connect to a wireless local area network (WLAN) using radio waves.

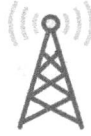

INDEX